Atlas of Hemofiltration

Commissioning Editor: Paul Fam
Project Development Manager: Sheila Black
Project Manager: Scott Millar
Designer: Jayne Jones
Illustration Manager: Mick Ruddy

Atlas of Hemofiltration

Rinaldo Bellomo MBBS (Hons), MD, FRACP, FCCP
Assistant Professor of Medicine
Department of Intensive Care,
Austin & Repatriation Medical Centre,
Melbourne, Victoria
Australia

Ian Baldwin RN, MN, BApp Science-Nursing Ed
Clinical Educator
Department of Intensive Care,
Austin & Repatriation Medical Centre,
Melbourne, Victoria
Australia

Claudio Ronco MD
Director, CRRT Program
Division of Nephrology,
San Bortolo Hospital,
Vicenza,
Italy

Thomas Golper MD
Professor of Medicine
Division of Nephrology,
Vanderbilt University,
Nashville, Tennessee,
USA

with the technical assistance of Flaviano Ghiotto, IP

W.B. SAUNDERS

LONDON • EDINBURGH • NEW YORK • PHILADELPHIA • ST LOUIS • SYDNEY • TORONTO 2002

WB SAUNDERS
An imprint of Harcourt Publishers Limited

© Harcourt Publishers Limited 2002

WB is a registered trademark of Harcourt Publishers Limited

The right of Rinaldo Bellomo, Ian Baldwin, Claudio Ronco
and Thomas Golper to be identified as authors of this work
has been asserted by them in accordance with the Copyright,
Designs and Patents Act 1988

First published 2002

ISBN 0 7020 2504 6

British Library Cataloguing in Publication Data
A catalogue record for this book is available from the British
Library

Library of Congress Cataloging in Publication Data
A catalog record for this book is available from the Library of
Congress

Note
Medical knowledge is constantly changing. As new
information becomes available, changes in treatment,
procedures, equipment and the use of drugs become
necessary. The editors/authors/contributors and the
publishers have taken care to ensure that the information
given in this text is accurate and up to date. However, readers
are strongly advised to confirm that the information, especially
with regard to drug usage, complies with the latest legislation
and standards of practice.

Existing UK nomenclature is changing to the system of
Recommended International Nonproprietary Names (rINNs).
Until the UK names are no longer in use, these more familiar
names are used in this book in preference to rINNs, details
of which may be obtained from the British National
Formulary.

The
publisher's
policy is to use
**paper manufactured
from sustainable forests**

Printed by the RDC Group in China

Contents

Contributors

Ian Baldwin, RN MN BApp Science–Nursing Ed
Clinical Educator
Department of Intensive Care
Austin & Repatriation Medical Centre
Heidelberg
Australia

Corrado Bellini
RanD s r l
Cavezzo (MO)
Italy

Rinaldo Bellomo, MBBS MD FRACP FCCP
Assistant Professor of Medicine (Intensive Care)
Department of Intensive Care
Austin & Repatriation Medical Centre
Heidelberg
Australia

Nicholas Bridge, RN
Department of Intensive Care
Austin & Repatriation Medical Centre
Heidelberg
Australia

Tania Elderkin, RN
Department of Intensive Care
Austin & Repatriation Medical Centre
Heidelberg
Australia

Luciano Fecondini
Medica s r l
Medolla (MO)
Italy

Flaviano Ghiotto, IP
Nurse in Charge
Hemodialysis and CRRT Program
Ospedale San Bortolo
Vicenza
Italy

Thomas Golper, MD
Professor of Medicine
Vanderbilt University
Division of Nephrology
Nashville, TN
USA

Gerhard Marquart and Meg Blogg
Edwards Life sciences GmbH
Unterschleissheim
Germany

Anne Morrison, RN BN (Hons) PIC Cert
Clinical Nurse Consultant
Pediatric Intensive Care Unit
The Children's Hospital at
Westmead, NSW
Australia

Claudio Ronco, MD
Director
CRRT Program
Division of Nephrology
San Bortolo Hospital
Vicenza
Italy

Lynne Snyder
B. Braun Medical Inc.
Bethlehem, PA
USA

Ciro Tetta
Bellco Spa
Mirandola (MO)
Italy

Barry Wilkins, MD MA MRCP(UK) FCRPCH FRACP
DCH (Lond)
Senior Staff Specialist
Pediatric Intensive Care Unit
The Children's Hospital at
Westmead, NSW
Australia

Preface

Continuous renal replacement therapy (CRRT) has gone from strength to strength over the last two decades. It started out as a simple therapy using arterio-venous access, high-flux filters and spontaneous ultrafiltration. This system developed close to 20 years ago, has undergone major changes. Modern CRRT has now become a veno-venous therapy with multiple methodologic variations (CVVH, CVVHD, CVVHDF) and an increasing array of technology. Despite this increase in sophistication, CRRT has become widespread throughout the world as the therapy of choice for artificial renal support in the ICU. In Australia, it is used in preference to intermittent hemodialysis for >90% of acute renal failure patients in the ICU. In Europe, approximately 50% of patients with ARF of critical illness are now also treated with CRRT. In America, the use of CRRT is also growing rapidly.

As the technology of CRRT becomes more complex and the machines more sophisticated, increasing demand is placed on practitioners to understand the principles and practicalities of CRRT. It has also become important for nephrologists, intensivists, dialysis nurses and ICU nurses to become familiar with a variety of machines. Such practitioners who work at the 'coal face' of patient care, must know how to prime and operate CRRT machines and how to trouble-shoot when the conduction of CRRT is not as smooth as planned. They must understand the tricks and traps of circuit diagnostics in order to make the correct diagnosis of what might be wrong and then implement the correct technical 'therapy'. They must understand the subtleties of anticoagulation and its drawbacks. They must have an appreciation of the strategies available for the prolongation of filter life. They must understand the reason for different approaches to vascular access and be able to identify access dysfunction or failure and treat it correctly. They must understand the clinical indications for CRRT, its extraordinary flexibility and usefulness in the ICU as a temperature controller, a volume controller, an acid–base homeostat and a tonicity regulator, as well as its limitations.

It is with these issues in mind that we have produced this *Atlas of Hemofiltration*. Our intention is to give nephrologists, intensivists, dialysis nurses and intensive care nurses a tool to increase their ability to effectively implement and conduct a CRRT program in their institution. By combining practical advice, clinical observations, technological information, step by step illustrations and discussion of basic therapeutic principles, we hope to have achieved our aims. The goal of our work is and remains one and one only: to give our patients the best chance to survive.

Rinaldo Bellomo
Ian Baldwin
Claudio Ronco
Thomas Golper
2001

Dedication

To all physicians and nurses who have embraced continuous renal replacement therapy in an effort to give their critically ill patients the best form of artificial renal support.

An Introduction to Continuous Renal Replacement Therapy

Rinaldo Bellomo and Claudio Ronco

Introduction

Continuous hemofiltration was first described more than 20 years ago[1]. Over this period, it has undergone remarkable changes, which have made it one of the great success stories of intensive care medicine. As we enter a new century and reach hemofiltration's 20th birthday, it is useful to understand its principles and evolution. The nephrologist, intensivist, dialysis nurse and critical care nurse will benefit from understanding the reasons for such evolution and from appreciating the present status of continuous hemofiltration (or, as more recently named, continuous renal replacement therapy – CRRT). They will also benefit from becoming aware of the trends in thinking and practice that appear likely to bring about further modifications and transformations in this novel form of extracorporeal therapy. This introduction is aimed at providing an overview of the principles of renal replacement therapy, a description of the evolution in its application in the intensive care unit (ICU), an update of recent research in this area and an insight into what the future may bring.

The principles

If physicians or nurses want to understand the development of CRRT, they need to understand the principles of blood purification by means of semi-permeable membranes. First, one must appreciate the mechanisms of fluid and solute transport across such membranes. They are diffusion, convection and ultrafiltration. During *diffusion* (Figure 1.1) the movement of solute depends on its statistical tendency to reach the same concentration in the available distribution space on each side of the membrane. The

practical result is the passage of solutes from the compartment with the highest concentration to the compartment with the least concentration[1]. During *convection* (Figure 1.2), on the other hand, the movement of solute across a semi-permeable membrane takes place in conjunction with significant amounts of ultrafiltration and water transfer across the membrane. Stated in another way, during convection, solute is 'carried'

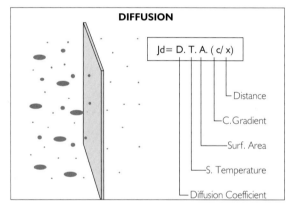

Figure 1.1: Illustration summarizing the principle of diffusion. Jd indicates diffusive movement.

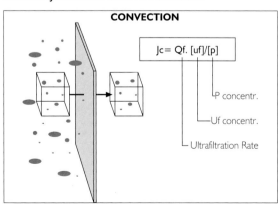

Figure 1.2: Illustration summarizing the principle of convection. Jc indicates convective movement.

by solvent, as the solvent (water) is pushed across the membrane (a process called ultrafiltration) in response to a transmembrane pressure gradient. Clearly, the porosity of the membrane is a major determinant of which solutes are removed during any blood purification therapy. In some situations, the two modes of solute transport occur simultaneously and in near equal proportions (hemodiafiltration)[2]. Ultrafiltration is a process by which plasma water and crystalloids are separated from whole blood across a semi-permeable membrane in response to a transmembrane pressure gradient. The process is governed by the following formula:

$$Qf = Km \times TMP$$

Where **Qf** is the ultrafiltration rate (ml/min), **Km** is the membrane ultrafiltration coefficient (derived from the ratio Qf/TMP and expressed in (ml/h) × (m²/mmHg) and **TMP** is the transmembrane pressure gradient generated by the pressures on both sides of the membrane. The hydrostatic pressure in the blood compartment is, of course, dependent on blood flow. The greater the blood flow rate, the greater the transmembrane pressure. Therefore, in a spontaneous ultrafiltration system based on convective clearance, measures that maximize blood flow rate will maximize ultrafiltrate production and solute clearance. Equally, measures that increase the negative pressure on the ultrafiltrate compartment of the membrane will generally also increase ultrafiltration, as will measures that decrease the oncotic pressure of plasma (pre-dilution, i.e. the administration of replacement fluid before the filter). As ultrafiltration proceeds and plasma water is ultrafiltered, hydrostatic pressure is lost and oncotic pressure is gained[3]. Thus, if the filter is long enough, a condition of filtration/pressure equilibrium is achieved where the oncotic pressure is equal to or greater than transmembrane pressure and ultrafiltration ceases. In modern filters, however, this is rarely, if ever, the case.

The relationship between transmembrane pressure and oncotic pressure will determine the filtration fraction, i.e. the fraction of plasma water that is removed from blood during hemofiltration. The optimal filtration fraction for

patients with a hematocrit of approximately 30% is in the range of 20–25%. This degree of filtration prevents excessive hemoconcentration at the filter outlet, which, in turn, would promote filter clotting.

Ultrafiltration control can also be obtained by applying a negative pressure generated by a pump (volumetric or peristaltic) to the ultrafiltration side of the filtering membrane. If such pressure is applied, attention must be paid to the maintenance of a safe filtration fraction. It is worth noting that with modern filters, the initial effect of controlling ultrafiltration is to retard it and to generate a positive pressure on the ultrafiltrate side of the hemofilter. Thus, TMP is initially decreased. As the filter fibers start to 'foul', a negative pressure becomes necessary to maintain a constant ultrafiltration rate. It is important, especially if one is using hemofiltration pumps to achieve continuous plasmafiltration, that transmembrane pressure must be kept within the range specified by the manufacturers. If this is not done, filter clotting becomes likely and membrane rupture may occur.

Blood purification technology

The membrane

Membranes employed during RRT can be divided into two categories: cellulose-based and synthetic membranes[4].

Cellulose-based membranes. These membranes (Cuprophan, Hemophan, Cellulose Acetate) are generally considered 'low flux' membranes, i.e. membranes with a permeability coefficient to water (K_m) <10 ml/h × mmHg/m². Cellulose-based membranes are very thin (5 to 15 μm of wall thickness) and have a symmetric structure with uniform porosity. They are strongly hydrophilic.

Synthetic membranes. These membranes (Polysulfone, Polyamide, Polyacrylonitrile, Polymethylmethacrylate) are high flux membranes with a K_m >30 ml/h × mmHg/m². Wall thickness ranges from 40–100 μm with an asymmetric structure composed of an inner skin layer and a surrounding sponge layer. Synthetic membranes have large pores (10–30 000 daltons) and are hydrophobic. They also have high sieving coefficients for solutes in a wide range of molecular weights and are much more suitable for convective treatments. Convective high filtration rates always take place when these membranes are used and such extracorporeal RRT is not adequately defined by the use of the term 'hemodialysis'. Such treatment is more appropriately called '**hemofiltration**' in the absence of diffusive clearance, '**hemodiafiltration**' if replacement solution is needed in addition to diffusive clearance or '**high flux dialysis**' if a filtration-backfiltration mechanism is present and no replacement is required[5].

Vascular access and the extracorporeal circuit

Extracorporeal blood treatments also require vascular access and a specific extracorporeal circuit design. Two different approaches are in use for extracorporeal treatments: arterio-venous and veno-venous mode.

Arterio-venous mode: In this system, the arterio-venous pressure gradient of the patient is the driving force moving blood through the circuit[6]. An artery and a vein are cannulated with large bore catheters (size 10–14 Fr) and no blood pumps are utilized. Maximal care is taken to avoid unnecessary resistance along the length of the circuit. Therefore, large and short catheters, short blood lines and short filters are utilized in this case. The determinants of ultrafiltration are different from those generally considered in pumped circulations. Hematocrit, plasma protein concentration (oncotic pressure) and the distance between the filter and the ultrafiltrate collection system become critical factors. In this system, blood flow generally ranges from 50–150 ml/min. In some patients, vascular access may require the surgical construction of a Scribner shunt. Blood flows under these circumstances tend to be between 60–80 ml/min. In the opinion of the authors, this system carries an excess of vascular access-related morbidity and should only be used in the absence of peristaltic pump availability.

Veno-venous mode: This type of circulation requires a roller pump in the prefilter line segment and a drip chamber in the line returning the blood from the filter[7]. Typically, a single central vein is cannulated with a double lumen catheter. Such double lumen catheters are now available on the market, are of size 11.5 to 13.5 Fr and can be easily inserted percutaneously by the Seldinger technique. In critically ill patients, the site of choice for the insertion of a double lumen catheter is usually determined by the patients' underlying disease and various clinical considerations. For example, patients with coagulopathy are more safely managed with a femoral catheter because the femoral site is more amenable to compression in case of inadvertent arterial puncture. The common feature of all double lumen catheters is the presence of a lumen that functions as the 'arterial' or outflow limb of the circuit and of a lumen which functions as the 'venous' or inflow limb of the circuit. Blood lines can be longer than in A-V circuits and a pressure measurement is required before the pump and after the filter to ensure safe use of the blood pump and to avoid any damage to the cannulated vein. In this system, blood flow can usually be kept between 150–200 ml/min.

Vascular access is discussed in detail in Chapter 16

The delivery of replacement fluid and dialysate

In continuous hemodialysis and hemodiafiltration, a dialysate flow rate from 10–30 ml/min is generally considered sufficient. Dialysate delivery can be performed by gravity, by means of infusion pumps or by a roller pump. The same system can be applied to the dialysate and ultrafiltrate outlet line in order to achieve fluid control. In continuous high flux dialysis, a couple of pumps are required to maintain effective ultrafiltration control. Sterile dialysate can be recirculated or run in single pass. In those treatments where replacement solution is needed to maintain patient fluid balance (CAVH-CVVH-CAVHDF-CVVHDF (nomenclature is discussed in detail in Chapter 2)), substitution fluid can be infused both in postdilutional or predilutional mode. The use of pumps to control fluid replacement and removal is increasing as it offers the advantage of decreasing nursing workload. It is otherwise possible to operate a spontaneous system of filtration with replacement being based on frequent (hourly) measurements of ultrafiltrate production. Sterile replacement/dialysate fluids for hemofiltration are now commercially available and contain different buffers such as bicarbonate, lactate and acetate.

Anticoagulation

All forms of RRT expose blood to contact with a non-biologic surface and therefore activate the clotting cascade. Anticoagulation of the extracorporeal circuit is thus desirable and, at times, necessary if one wants to perform RRT safely and effectively. There are several approaches to anticoagulation during RRT and they are discussed in detail in Chapter 14.

Initiating and maintaining RRT

Many clinicians feel that renal replacement therapy is best initiated early in the course of the patient's illness. They believe that it is physiologically unsound and clinically dangerous to wait for any of the complications of uremia to develop before dialytic therapy is undertaken. Now that CRRT is available and hemodynamic instability can be avoided, there is little morbidity associated with initiating RRT early, even in the sickest of patients. There are no scientific studies, however, to help the physician decide when to start RRT. Time-honored criteria are simply descriptors of uremic complications such as pulmonary edema, severe fluid overload, hyperkalemia, uncontrolled uremia, uremic complications and severe uncontrolled metabolic acidosis. Attempts are usually made to prevent such complications by means of various conservative maneuvers (diuretics, medical treatments of hyperkalemia, bicarbonate administration, fluid restrictions and nutritional restrictions). When they fail, treatment is escalated to intermittent hemodialysis (IHD) or other forms of renal replacement. A different and more aggressive approach to the above problems, however, has recently been advocated in the ICU, where maintenance of homeostasis and prevention of complications are an important therapeutic goal[8]. According to such an approach, prevention is superior to treatment, early intervention is desirable and CRRT offers the ideal form of RRT for such an approach. According to a more prevention-based approach, different criteria for initiating RRT in the ICU should now be considered (Table 1.1).

Table 1.1: Modern indications for initiating RRT in adult critically ill patients

1. Oliguria (urine output <200 ml/12 h)
2. Anuria or extreme oliguria (urine output <50 ml/12 h)
3. Hyperkalemia ([K^+] >6.5 mmol/l and rising)
4. Severe acidemia (pH <7.1)
5. Azotemia ([urea] >30 mmol/l or [creat] >300 µmol/l)
6. Pulmonary edema
7. Uremic encephalopathy
8. Uremic pericarditis
9. Uremic neuropathy or myopathy
10. Severe dysnatremia ([Na^+] >160 or <115 mmol/l)
11. Hyperthermia
12. Drug overdose with filterable toxin (Lithium, Vancomycin, Procainamide etc.)
13. Anasarca
14. Diuretic-resistant cardiac failure
15. Imminent/ongoing massive blood product administration

NB: The presence of one of the above criteria is sufficient to initiate RRT. The simultaneous presence of two of these criteria makes the prompt initiation of RRT highly desirable. The presence of three criteria makes the prompt initiation of RRT mandatory. In all of these cases, CRRT is the preferred approach.

Once RRT has been instituted, there is no scientifically established biochemical or clinical measure of so-called dialytic adequacy. However, most clinicians using CRRT seek to maintain a urea concentration of at least <30 mmol/l and preferably <25 mmol/l. Normalization of electrolytes, phosphate and calcium is also pursued. The ideal therapy should achieve these goals with a minimum of morbidity and at reasonable cost. The ideal dialysis dose in critically ill patients, however, remains unclear and we still have little information on the relationship between the 'dose' of dialysis and outcomes in acute renal failure (ARF). Early randomized, controlled trials comparing intensive dialysis to less aggressive treatment were of insufficient statistical power to come to a conclusion, although some positive trends were reported. Moreover, the gap between dialysis prescribed and dialysis delivered may be in excess of 20% or more in end stage renal disease (ESRD). It may be even more pronounced with ARF due to hemodynamic instability; reduced blood flow; shortened dialysis time because of scheduled procedures or diagnostic tests; and suboptimal vascular access. Despite these caveats, the preliminary reports from Paganini et al[9] are worth noting. In the first report, the authors examined the influence of dialytic modality (IHD vs. CRRT, not randomly allocated) in 856 critically ill patients with ARF. Among the 280 patients treated with IHD, there was no significant association between prescribed dialysis dose and the odds of death. Mortality was strongly associated with severity of illness and comorbidity. In a more recent report, however, patients were categorized into risk quartiles based on an institution-specific severity of illness and comorbidity score[10]. Dialysis dose was not associated with mortality at either extreme of risk (very low or very high risk). However, mortality was reduced in intermediate-risk patients treated with more intensive dialysis, defined as a urea reduction ratio in excess of 58% in patients on IHD, and a time-averaged urea concentration below 45 mg/dl in patients treated with CRRT. Renal recovery and other outcomes were not reported. Schiffl et al[11] recently reported the preliminary results of a randomized clinical trial. In this trial, 72 patients with ARF were randomized to either daily or alternate day IHD. Mortality was significantly reduced in the daily IHD group (21% vs. 47%). These data are provocative, but require confirmation elsewhere. However, based on data derived from ESRD patients and limited data in ARF, it can be said, in general, that more dialysis is better. Of course, the use of CRRT can solve all problems of dialysis delivery and Kt/V calculations. CRRT can always maintain steady and high level control of uremia 24 hours per day.

Controversies in the choice of RRT in the ICU

There are no randomized controlled trials to guide the clinician in their choice of the best form of RRT for a given critically ill patient. Not surprisingly, in the absence of such a trial, there is much controversy and disagreement concerning the choice of RRT in the ICU. In the adult population, however, peritoneal dialysis is now used infrequently in developed countries. This lack of application is due to several factors that include insufficient solute clearance[12], limited control of hyperkalemia, a high incidence of peritonitis, poor fluid removal, unpredictable fluctuations in glycemia, abdominal leaks and respiratory dysfunction. Because of these factors, the major controversy pertains to the preferential use of CRRT vs. IHD. This controversy has generally divided practitioners across national or regional lines with Australian and European intensivists increasingly adopting CRRT and with American nephrologists choosing to remain with IHD. Although this controversy is likely to remain unresolved, some observations (see below) may assist the intensivist in appreciating the pros and cons of the options available. The first observation is that hemodialysis is associated with several clinically important complications (Table 1.2). The most important of these complications in critically ill patients with multiorgan dysfunction is the development of hypotension. Such hypotension is most severe in those patients that are most cardiovascularly unstable[13]. The physiological cost of such hypotension is clinically significant, as IHD may precipitate ischemia in specific organs such as the recovering kidneys, which have temporarily lost pressure-flow autoregulation. Such ischemia can be seen histologically as fresh ischemic lesions occurring with each episode of IHD[14]. Such lesions delay renal recovery. Additional to hemodynamic instability, the other major concern associated with episodic fluid removal with IHD is the intermittent fluid overload that occurs between treatments. In the extreme case, this can be unacceptable, as is the case for oliguric patients with acute respiratory distress syndrome

---

Table 1.2: Major complications of intermittent hemodialysis.

Systemic hypotension
Arrhythmia
Hypoxemia
Hemorrhage
Infection
Line-related complications (e.g. pneumothorax)
Seizure/dialysis disequilibrium
Pyrogen reaction or hemolysis
? Delay in recovery of renal function

(ARDS) who will not easily tolerate excess extravascular water. CRRT is the obvious choice in such patients. Indeed CRRT may also improve respiratory function in patients with multiorgan failure and acute lung injury. An important practical benefit of CRRT is its ability to continuously remove as much water and sodium as desired. This ability particularly impacts on patient nutrition, which can be delivered without restriction[15]. The importance of feeding the critically ill adequately has been borne out by studies demonstrating a correlation between mortality and a progressive calorie deficit as well as an association between patient morbidity and cumulative protein intake. The advantage of CRRT is that uremic control can always be achieved and maintained even in septic patients while providing sufficient nutritional support. When compared with IHD, both CAVHD and CVVHD are superior in delivering the required daily nutrients. It should also be noted that the daily loss of free amino acids during CRRT is similar to that seen during a 4-hour hemodialysis session, i.e. approximately 1–2 g N_2 or 10% of the usual daily intake. Lastly, it is worth remembering that CRRT also reduces energy expenditure by cooling the febrile patients and that no hormonal or trace element losses of significance take place during CRRT. Vitamin losses are also minimal, except for vitamin C, which is lost in amounts roughly equivalent to its recommended daily allowance. There are now several reports on the utility of hemofiltration in patients with heart failure that is resistant to diuretics. Such patients often respond well to continuous ultrafiltration with a rise in cardiac index, while avoiding a fall in arterial pressure. The hemodynamic improvement is mostly due to a change in preload, which optimizes myocardial contractility on the Starling curve. Many patients with congestive cardiac failure not responding to conventional therapy are now successfully treated in this way. The rationale of using a continuous therapy is to achieve a physiological, safe and progressive removal of fluid and solute. The cumulative clearance of urea and creatinine by a continuous method is superior (clinically and statistically) to that achieved by intermittent hemodialysis applied up to 4 times per week, even in septic patients. Indeed, IHD applied 6

times per week would be necessary to achieve the same uremic control seen with standard CRRT[16]. The net result is that, in practice, uremic control is clearly superior during CRRT[17].

Another disadvantage of the faster, diffusive clearance of solute with IHD is that it causes solute disequilibrium. Solute is thus extracted from the intravascular space by the dialyzer at a rate that is substantially faster than solute movement into blood from the intracellular and interstitial compartments. Such solute disequilibrium may be responsible for brain edema[18] and has even more pronounced ill effects in the critically ill; particularly those with increased intracranial pressure[19]. In high-risk patients, rapid solute movements may cause tonsillar herniation and death. CRRT, on the other hand, does not induce such surges in intracranial pressure and maintains cerebral perfusion pressure[19]. CRRT is therefore the treatment of choice in all patients with, or at risk of, cerebral edema.

Other practical considerations regarding differences between CRRT and IHD include thermal loss, anticoagulation, and patient mobilization. The ability to cool febrile patients may be beneficial as it is often accompanied by amelioration of tachycardia and vasodilatation. However, because this effect conceals some clinical signs of infection, the clinician should have a lower threshold for suspecting ongoing sepsis. Anticoagulation of the hemofiltration circuit with heparin is safe and adequate in the vast majority of patients. In those at risk of bleeding, various alternative approaches are used including low dose heparin, regional heparinization, low molecular weight heparin, prostacyclin, citrate and no anticoagulation. It is not uncommon that persisting difficulties with circuit clotting are due to problems with vascular access. This can occur irrespective of whether continuous or intermittent treatment is being employed. Overall, the need for anticoagulation does not pose a sufficient obstacle to the use of CRRT in contrast to IHD.

Despite the demonstrable physiological benefits of using CRRT in critically ill patients, some believe that, in the absence of a proven effect on mortality, IHD should be regarded as the standard approach. The difficulty, however, is that to demonstrate such a difference would require the randomization of more than a thousand patients in a multicenter study with standardization of other clinical management. Two attempts have been made to conduct such studies. Both have had difficulty with methodology, randomization and with recruitment of patients; neither has yet been published in full and neither has achieved conclusive results so far. Furthermore, it has been noted that as more ICUs change to using CRRT, such a trial will be harder to undertake.

Of all the patients in intensive care, those receiving RRT have the poorest prognosis and yet cost the most. It is therefore important to consider the costs of the treatment used in these patients including those of renal replacement and to relate them to the gains in life-years. Although the general principles of cost estimation apply throughout, they must be calculated for individual units to account for local factors such as salaries, costs of replacement or dialysate fluids, methods of anticoagulation and rates of depreciation of equipment purchased. One such costing analysis was carefully performed at Guy's hospital in London. The costs of the two methods were found to be very close with the IHD being only 6% cheaper[20]. CAVHD would be cheaper overall as a blood pump would not be required. In addition, recent data from a randomized, controlled trial show that complete renal recovery is significantly more common with CRRT than with IHD. This finding suggests that there may be hidden costs in association with an IHD-based approach.

Septic shock, multiorgan failure, ARF and renal replacement therapy

Many patients with ARF have severe sepsis, multiorgan dysfunction and a major systemic inflammatory response. In these patients, the blood purification achieved with CRRT may provide additional advantages that go beyond renal replacement therapy *per se* and move into the area of immunomodulation. In fact, the demonstrated ability that CRRT has to remove or adsorb putative mediators of organ dysfunction may represent yet another reason for its preferential application[21]. Recent investigations in

animals and humans suggest that, if hemofiltration is to have an additional role in the management of sepsis, the rate of plasma water exchange will have to be increased[22,23]. The effect of CRRT in sepsis may increase survival in patients with sepsis-associated ARF[24]. In response to these developments, investigators are now seeking to augment the blood purification efficacy of CRRT in a direction more clearly aimed at immune system modulation. Initial experience is accumulating in the treatment of severe sepsis with organ dysfunction using high volume hemofiltration[25] or coupled plasmafiltration with adsorption[26] (Figures 1.1 and 1.2). Such experience suggests that, at the very least, these more aggressive approaches to blood purification can decrease the need for vasopressor therapy during septic shock. More recently, the concept that convective CRRT in the form of CVVH is more effective at lowering circulating levels of soluble inflammatory mediators than diffusive CRRT in the form of CVVHD has been tested in a randomized, controlled study[27]. This elegant study demonstrated that for equal amounts of dialysate/replacement fluid administration rate, convective therapy achieves lower serum TNF concentrations than diffusive therapy. The findings of this study lend further support to the preferential use of convective therapy.

Another area where hemofiltration is proving remarkably useful is the control of fluid balance in patients requiring extracorporeal membrane oxygenation for cardiogenic shock after cardiac surgery. These patients often require massive amounts of clotting factors, which can only be given safely in the presence of continuous hemofiltration. Under such circumstances, fluid can be removed as the clotting factors are being administered and the development of ARDS/pulmonary edema can be prevented while the bleeding is controlled. Under such circumstances, hemofiltration can be performed without any need for circuit anticoagulation. We have also used hemofiltration to treat patients with ARDS in whom attempts to induce a negative fluid balance with loop diuretics result in a water diuresis but not a salt diuresis. In such patients, hypernatremia develops and extravascular lung water is not decreased. Continuous hemofiltration under these circumstances achieves normalization of serum sodium levels and the removal of extravascular water while maintaining full hemodynamic stability. This process often achieves substantial improvements in gas exchange and lung compliance.

Conclusion

In conclusion, the clinician taking care of critically ill patients with multiorgan failure including severe ARF needs to be aware of many issues. He or she also needs to understand the implications of recent changes in the area of renal replacement technology[28]. It is likely that the application of CRRT will continue to grow in intensive care units around the world and that the intensivist will be called upon to play an increasingly important role in its prescription and execution. Furthermore, as the knowledge base in this area of medicine expands, physicians involved in 'critical care nephrology'[29] should develop a unique level of expertise in order to improve patient outcomes. Artificial renal support remains a large component of the practice of critical care and may expand to the adjunctive management of septic shock. The critical care physician can no longer partly neglect it or completely delegate its prescription and execution to others. In order to move forward, attention needs to be focused on this component of the care of critically ill patients. Co-operation between nephrologists and intensivists needs to be strongly promoted. Only then will we see the mortality of these patients significantly decline.

References

1. Kolff WJ. The artificial kidney – past and future. *Circulation* 1957; 15: 285
2. Henderson LW, Lilley JJ, Ford CA, Stone RA. Hemodiafiltration. *J Dial* 1977; 1: 211–217.
3. Ronco C, Orlandini G, Brendolan A, Lupi A, La Greca G. Enhancement of convective transport by internal filtration in a modified experimental hemodialyzer. *Kidney Int* 1998; 54: 979–985.
4. Konstantin P. Newer membranes: cuprophan versus polysulfone versus polyacrylonitrile. In: Bosch JP, ed. *Hemodialysis: High Efficiency Treatments. Contemporary Issues in Nephrology.* New York: Churchill Livingstone 1993; 27: 63–78.
5. Ronco C, Bellomo R. Continuous high-flux dialysis: an efficient renal replacement. In: Vincent JL, ed. 1996 *Yearbook of Intensive Care and Emergency Medicine.* Berlin: Springer-Verlag 1996, 690–698.
6. Lauer A, Saccaggi A, Ronco C, Belledonne M, Glabman S, Bosch JP. Continuous arteriovenous hemofiltration in the critically ill patient. *Ann Intern Med* 1983; 99: 455–460.
7. Bellomo R, Ronco C. Circulation of the continuous artificial kidney: Blood flow, pressures, clearances, and the search for the best. In Ronco C, Artigas A, Bellomo R (eds). *Circulation in Native and Artificial Kidneys.* Basel: S. Karger, 1997; 354–365.
8. Bellomo R, Ronco C. Acute renal failure in the intensive care unit: adequacy of dialysis and the case for continuous therapies. *Nephrol Dial Transplant* 1996; 11: 424–428.
9. Paganini EP, Tapolyai M, Goormastic M *et al.* Establishing a dialysis therapy/patient outcome link in intensive care unit acute dialysis for patients with acute renal failure. *Am J Kidney Dis* 1996; 28: S81–S89.
10. Paganini EP, Halstenberg WK, Goormastic M. Risk modeling in acute renal failure requiring dialysis: the introduction of a new model. *Clin Nephrol* 1996; 46: 206–211.
11. Schiffl H, Lang SM, Konig A, Held E. Dose of intermittent hemodialysis and outcome of acute renal failure: a prospective randomized study. *J Am Soc Nephrol* 1997; 8: 290A.
12. Howdieshell TR, Blalock WE, Bowen PA, Hawkins ML, Hess C. Management of post-traumatic acute renal failure with peritoneal dialysis. *Am Surg* 1992; 6: 378–382.
13. Hakim RM, Wingard RL, Parker RA. Effect of the dialysis membrane in the treatment of patients with acute renal failure. *N Engl J Med* 1994; 331: 1338–1342.
14. Conger JD. Does hemodilaysis delay recovery from acute renal failure? *Semin Dial* 1990; 3: 146–148.
15. Bellomo R, Seacombe J, Daskalakis M *et al.* A prospective comparative study of moderate versus high protein intake for critically ill patients with acute renal failure. *Renal Failure* 1997; 19: 11–20.

16. Clark WR, Macias WL. Azotemia control by extracorporeal therapy in patients with acute renal failure. *New Horizons* 1995; 3: 688–698.

17. Ronco C. Continuous renal replacement therapies for the treatment of acute renal failure in intensive care patients. *Clin Nephrol* 1993; 40: 187–198.

18. La Greca G, Biasioli S, Chiaramonte S *et al*. Studies on brain density in hemodialysis and peritoneal dialysis. *Nephron* 1982; 31: 146–150.

19. Davenport A. The management of renal failure in patients at risk of cerebral edema/hypoxia. *New Horizons* 1995; 3: 717–724.

20. Silvester W. Outcome studies of continuous renal replacement therapy in the intensive care unit. *Kidney Int* 1998; 53; Suppl 66: S138–S141.

21. Bellomo R. Continuous hemofiltration as blood purification in sepsis. *New Horizons* 1995; 3: 732–738.

22. Grootendorst AF, van Bommel EFH, van der Hoven B *et al*. High-volume hemofiltration improves hemodynamics in endotoxin-induced shock in the pig. *J Crit Care* 1992; 7: 67–75.

23. Cole L, Bellomo R, Baldwin I. A randomized cross-over study of the hemodynamic effects of high volume hemofiltration in patients with septic shock. *Blood Purif* 1998; 16: 113–114.

24. Bellomo R, Farmer M, Wright C, Parkin G, Boyce N. Treatment of sepsis-associated severe acute renal failure with continuous hemodiafiltration: clinical experience and comparison with conventional dialysis. *Blood Purif* 1995; 13: 246–254.

25. Bellomo R, Cole L, Baldwin I, Ronco C. Preliminary experience with high-volume hemofiltration in human septic shock. *Kidney Int* 1998; 53; Suppl 66: S182–S185.

26. Tetta C, Cavaillon JM, Camussi G, Lonneman FG, Brendolan A, Ronco C. Continuous plasma filtration coupled with absorbents. *Kidney Int* 1998; 53; Suppl 66: S186–S189.

27. Kellum JA, Johnson JP, Kramer D, Palevsky P, Brady JJ, Pinsky MR. Diffusive vs. convective therapy: Effects on mediators of inflammation in patients with severe systemic inflammatory response syndrome. *Crit Care Med* 1998; 26: 1995–2000.

28. Bellomo R, Mehta R. Acute renal replacement in the intensive care unit: now and tomorrow. *New Horizons* 1995; 3: 760–767.

29. Ronco C, Bellomo R. Critical care nephrology: the time has come. *Nephrol Dial Transplant* 1998; 13: 264–267.

2

Nomenclature for Continuous Renal Replacement Therapy

Rinaldo Bellomo and Claudio Ronco

Introduction

Continuous hemofiltration has become more widespread and more information is disseminated in this field of medicine. It has also become quite important that an agreement upon nomenclature should be developed so that it is clear to all what therapy is being applied to patients (Convective? Diffusive? Mixed? Veno-venous? Arterio-venous? etc.). Such clarity of description will hopefully help practitioners communicate more effectively as well as help the science of CRRT develop more rapidly. What is presented below is a summary of the consensus nomenclature agreed upon at the 1996 International CRRT Conference[1].

Techniques and their nomenclature

It is important for the critical care physician to understand and appreciate the differences between renal replacement therapies and the reasons for the relatively complex nomenclature that surrounds them. The following definitions reflect the principles and technical requirements of the various types of RRTs as recently agreed upon during a consensus conference[1].

Hemodialysis (HD)
This term defines a prevalently diffusive treatment in which blood and dialysate are circulated in countercurrent mode and a low permeability, cellulose-based membrane is employed. The ultrafiltration rate is approximately equal to the scheduled weight loss. This treatment can be performed intermittently (Intermittent Haemodialysis – IHD), e.g. 4 hours three times per week, daily (2–4 hours) or continuously, both in arterio-venous or veno-venous mode (CAVHD-CVVHD).

Peritoneal dialysis (PD)
This term refers to a predominantly diffusive treatment where blood, circulating along the capillaries of the peritoneal membrane, is exposed to dialysate. Access is obtained by the insertion of a peritoneal catheter, which allows the abdominal instillation of dialysate. Solute and water movement is achieved by means of variable concentration and tonicity gradients generated by the dialysate. This treatment can be performed intermittently or continuously.

Hemofiltration (HF)
This term defines an essentially convective treatment with highly permeable membranes. The ultrafiltrate produced is replaced completely or in part by a sterile solution of water and electrolytes. Blood purification and fluid control is thus achieved. Any net fluid loss will result from the difference between ultrafiltration and reinfusion rates (no dialysate is used). This treatment can be performed intermittently (30 l/session three times per week), daily (10–30 l exchange) or continuously, both in arterio-venous or veno-venous mode (CAVH or CVVH) (12–30 l of plasma water exchange/day)[2].

Hemodiafiltration (HDF)
This term defines a treatment in which diffusion and convection are combined utilizing a highly permeable membrane. Blood and dialysate are circulated as in hemodialysis but typically an ultrafiltration rate in excess of the scheduled weight loss is produced. To achieve fluid balance, a sterile solution of water and electrolytes is reinfused into the patient at an adequate rate. This treatment can be performed intermittently (3–4 hours at 9–15 l exchange/session three times per week), daily (3 hours and 9 l exchange)

or continuously, both in arterio-venous or veno-venous mode (CAVHDF–CVVHDF).

High flux dialysis (HFD)

This term describes a treatment that utilizes highly permeable membranes in conjunction with an ultrafiltration control system. Blood and dialysate are circulated as in hemodialysis, but due to the high permeability coefficient of the membrane, ultrafiltration would exceed the required patient weight loss. Therefore, a positive pressure is applied to the dialysate compartment to reduce the amount of ultrafiltration and to avoid the need for replacement solution. Due to the peculiar structure of hollow fiber dialyzers, filtration takes place in the proximal part of the filter, whilst backfiltration occurs in the distal part of the filter. Diffusion and convection, therefore, are still combined. The high filtration rate, which occurs in the proximal part of the dialyzer, is masked by backfiltration in the distal part. Replacement is avoided as it occurs inside the filter by the mechanism of backfiltration. Such backfiltration implies that, during HFD, dialysate must be sterile and pyrogen free[3].

Ultrafiltration (UF)

This term defines a treatment in which fluid removal is the main target of therapy. Highly permeable filters are utilized and fluid is removed from the body without providing any replacement solution. UF can be performed intermittently or daily, and a maximum of 3 l per session is generally removed in a period of 4–6 hours. In clinical practice, ultrafiltration has also been used in sequence with hemodialysis to improve cardiovascular tolerance. In critically ill patients, it can also be performed continuously at very low filtration rates (1–2 ml/min) with or without the addition of dialysate (SCUF or SCUF-D) to remove edema fluid. Both arterio-venous and veno-venous modes can be used.

Plasmapheresis (PF)

This term describes a treatment which uses peculiar plasmafilters. In these filters, the molecular weight cut-off of the membrane is much higher than that of hemofilters. Plasma as a whole is filtered and blood is reconstituted by the infusion of plasma products such as fresh frozen plasma, albumin or other fluids. This treatment is performed in an attempt to remove proteins or protein bound solutes that cannot be removed by simple hemofiltration.

Hemoperfusion (HP)

This term describes a form of treatment in which blood is circulated on a bed of coated charcoal powder to remove solutes by adsorption. The technique is specifically indicated in cases of poisoning or intoxication with agents that can be effectively removed by charcoal such as theophylline. This treatment causes frequent platelet and protein fraction depletion and therefore is utilized only in specific cases under intensive and continuous monitoring.

Abbreviations
Qb = blood flow rate
Qd = dialysate flow rate
Qf = ultrafiltrate flow rate

Slow Continuous Ultrafiltration
(arterio-venous or veno-venous)

Qb = 100–250 ml/min Qf = 2–10 ml/min

Abbreviation: SCUF (A–V SCUF or VVSCULF)

Technique where blood is driven through a highly permeable filter via an extracorporeal circuit in arterio-venous or veno-venous mode. The ultrafiltrate produced during membrane transit is not replaced and it corresponds to the patient weight loss (Figure 2.1)

Used only for fluid control in fluid overloaded patients

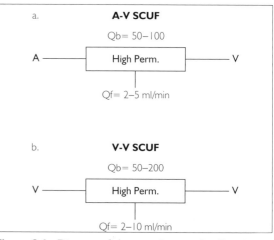

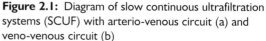

Figure 2.1: Diagram of slow continuous ultrafiltration systems (SCUF) with arterio-venous circuit (a) and veno-venous circuit (b)

Continuous hemofiltration

(arterio-venous or veno-venous)

Qb = 100–300 ml/min   Qf = 10–33 ml/min

Abbreviation: CAVH or CVVH

Technique whereby blood is driven through a highly permeable filter via an extracorporeal circuit in arterio-venous or veno-venous mode. The ultrafiltrate produced during membrane transit is replaced in part or completely to achieve blood purification and volume control. Ultrafiltration is in excess of patient's desired weight loss and replacement fluid is needed (Figure 2.2).

Clearance for all solute is convective and equals ultrafiltration rate

Continuous hemodialysis

(arterio-venous or veno-venous)

Qb = 80–200 ml/min Qf = 1–2 ml/min
Qd = 10–33 ml/min

Abbreviation: CAVHD or CVVHD

Technique whereby blood is driven through a low permeability dialyzer and a countercurrent flow of dialysate is delivered on the dialysate compartment. The ultrafiltrate produced during membrane transit corresponds to patient's weight loss. Solute clearance is mainly diffusive. Replacement solution is not needed (Figure 2.3).

Efficiency is limited to small solutes only

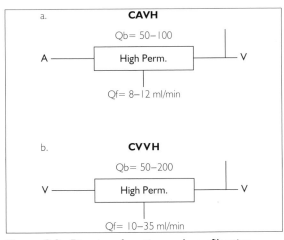

Figure 2.2: Diagram of continuous hemofiltration circuits with arterio-venous (CAVH) hemofiltration (a) and veno-venous hemofiltration (CVVH) (b).

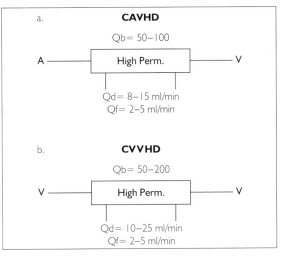

Figure 2.3: Diagram of continuous hemodialysis circuits with (a) arterio-venous circuit (CAVHD) and (b) veno-venous circuit (CVVHD).

Continuous hemodiafiltration

(arterio-venous or veno-venous)

Qb = 100–300 ml/min Qf = 8–15 ml/min
Qd = 10–33 ml/min

Abbreviation: CAVHDF or CVVHDF

Technique whereby blood is driven through a highly permeable dialyzer and a countercurrent flow of dialysis solution is delivered on the dialysate compartment. The ultrafiltrate produced during membrane transit is in excess of the patient's desired weight loss. Solute clearance is both diffusive and convective. Replacement solution needed to maintain fluid balance (Figure 2.4).

Efficiency is extended from small to larger molecules

Further definitions

Diffusion
A term that describes a type of solute transport across a semi-permeable membrane generated by a concentration gradient. Such solute has a statistical tendency to reach the same concentration in the available space on both sides of the membrane. Thus, molecules move from the compartment with the highest concentration to the one with the lowest. Diffusion is proportional to gradient, temperature, surface area, and solute diffusivity. It is inversely proportional to membrane thickness.

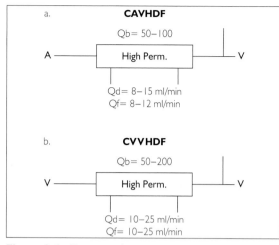

Figure 2.4: Diagram of a continuous hemodiafiltration system with (a) arterio-venous circuit (CAVHDF) and (b) veno-venous circuit (CVVHDF).

Convection

A term that describes a process by which solutes are transported across a semi-permeable membrane together with solvent by means of a filtration mechanism (solvent drag) in response to a transmembrane pressure gradient. Convection depends on filtration rate, membrane permeability and concentration of solute in plasma water.

Ultrafiltration

In renal replacement therapy, this term describes the process by which plasma water and filterable solutes are separated from whole blood across a semi-permeable membrane in response to a transmembrane pressure.

Ultrafiltrate

The plasma water and solutes produced during ultrafiltration.

Dialysate

The synthetic, uremic solute-free solution administered into the dialysate compartment of the filter/dialyzer in order to achieve diffusive solute clearance.

Diafiltrate

The plasma water and ultrafiltered solutes plus effluent dialysate produced during hemodiafiltration.

Arterio-venous (AV) circuit

A term describing the arterial and venous vascular access and the associated tubing necessary to carry blood into and out of the hemofilter and back to the patient.

Veno-venous (VV) circuit

A term describing the central venous vascular access and associated tubing carrying blood into and out of the hemofilter and back to the patient.

Pre-dilution

The administration of replacement fluid into the circuit before the filter.

Post-dilution

The administration of replacement fluid into the circuit after the filter.

Ultrafiltration control system

A technique whereby ultrafiltrate production is regulated by a pump applied to the ultrafiltration tubing.

Backfiltration

Flux of dialysate from its compartment into the blood in response to a local negative transmembrane pressure gradient. This process typically occurs in the presence of ultrafiltration control systems during therapy carried out with hollow fiber, high-flux membranes.

References

1. Bellomo R, Ronco C, Mehta RL. Nomenclature for continuous renal replacement therapy. *Am J Kidney Dis* 1996; 28: S2–S7.
2. Ronco C, Bellomo R. Continuous renal replacement therapy: evolution in technology and current nomenclature. *Kidney Int* 1998; 53: S160–S164.
3. Ronco C, Bellomo R. Continuous high-flux dialysis: an efficient renal replacement. In Vincent J-L (ed) *Yearbook of Intensive Care and Emergency Medicine.* Heidelberg: Springer-Verlag 1996; pp 690–696.

3

Solute Transport in CRRT

Thomas Golper

Introduction

The goals of blood cleansing vary by the conditions encountered in each individual situation. For example, after cardiac damage with hypotension CRRT may be utilized simply for salt and water removal. With renal failure and hypotension CRRT may be necessary for uremic solute removal as well as removal of salt and water. CRRT may be attempted in conditions where the exact nature of the solute is unclear, but the removal of some inflammatory mediators, vasodilators or myocardial depressants leads to an improvement in the overall clinical condition. This section will focus on general principles of solute removal and will describe unique conditions, such as those mentioned, wherein such principles are exemplified.

Diffusion

As a consequence of their thermal kinetic energy, solutes move through their solvent medium by Brownian motion, colliding into other particles, which alters their direction of otherwise random movement. Given enough time this type of motion results in the equal disperse distribution of these particles throughout the volume of the solvent solution. This dispersion process is called diffusion. The driving force for diffusion is the concentration of particles. A denser concentration of particles results in more frequent collisions (and direction changes) until the particles spread out or disperse. Particles tend to move from a higher to a lower concentration and thus the direction and speed of this particle dispersion is determined by the concentration gradient. In the plasma water of a uremic patient there is a higher concentration of species retained in uremia, such as urea, potassium, phosphates, and many more.

As will be discussed below synthetic semi-permeable membranes that separate plasma water (specifically, whole blood) from the cleansing solution dialysate, contain numerous pores that act as channels through which solutes diffuse and solvent flows. As stated above, diffusion occurs down a concentration gradient. The concentration of bicarbonate in dialysate is higher than the concentration in blood, so bicarbonate diffuses into the blood, while uremic retained solutes diffuse from blood to dialysate. Membranes with ideal diffusion properties act like water as a medium for diffusion; this is called hydrophilicity. A hydrophilic membrane soaks up water and acts like water, the ideal diffusion medium for dialysis. This is in contrast to some synthetic membranes, which are hydrophobic, do not absorb water, and have less ideal diffusion properties. These membranes possess other desirable qualities such as improved biocompatibility, protein adsorptive capacity, and increased hydraulic permeability. An increase in surface area (see below) can compensate for the poorer diffusivity of hydrophobic membranes.

Molecules or ions diffuse at an equal rate through an unrestricted medium. The membrane pores create a restricted medium such that the steric size of the molecule/ion slows down diffusion through the pore. For small solutes, arbitrarily defined as <500 daltons, membrane pores are essentially not restrictive to diffusion. Above this size, the larger the molecule/ion, the slower the diffusion. Molecules/ions may act larger than their molecular weight because of their intense polarity and the consequential attraction of water molecules. The phosphate anion is a prime example of a species diffusing much more slowly than one would expect from its molecular weight.

The size of the pore becomes a factor slowing the rate of diffusion of molecules of middle molecular weights (500–5000 daltons) and large molecular weights (>5000 daltons). All membranes possess heterogeneity in pore sizes.

The flux of a membrane is not the same thing as pore size. Flux refers to the hydraulic permeability and convective transport (see below). Pore size plays a role in the removal of middle sized drugs such as aminoglycosides and vancomycin, and small peptides such as PTH, insulin, myoglobin and β_2-microglobin. The larger the pore, the greater (faster) the diffusion for these larger species.

The mass transfer diffusion co-efficient is the measure of the diffusivity of the species *and* membrane in question. One component of this measure is the surface area. The surface area is the point of contact between the two solutions on each side of the semi-permeable membrane, so the larger the contact urea, the greater (faster) the diffusion.

Since diffusion is highly dependent upon the concentration gradient, to maximize diffusion one must maintain maximum concentration gradients. To achieve this goal one desires high concentrations of uremic solute in the blood entering the dialyzer and the absence of the species in the dialysate. Furthermore, one desires that the flow rate of solute entering the dialyzer and the flow rate of dialysate entering the dialyzer be as high as possible. The goal is to achieve a concentration gradient of infinity. The fresh dialysate has a concentration of zero, and non-recirculated blood has a concentration as high as anywhere in the body. Thus, dialysate and blood inflow rates are maximized. In addition, the concentration gradient between blood and dialysate is best maximized by flowing the dialysate countercurrent to blood flow. Thus at the blood outlet, where uremic solutes are at their lowest concentration, the dialysate concentration of these solutes (at the dialysate inlet) is at its lowest. At the dialysate outlet, where uremic solutes are now present, the blood concentration is at its highest. By countercurrent flow there is always a steep concentration gradient and diffusion is maximally efficient.

If all of a solute is removed from the blood (100% extraction) by one passage through a dialyzer, the whole blood clearance is equal to the blood flow rate. In general, the goal in blood cleansing is to maximize blood clearance or maximize net solute removal, rather than have a high extraction ratio. Total blood clearance can never exceed blood flow rate. At best, clearance can equal blood flow rate.

If dialysate exiting the dialyzer is saturated with solute, i.e. the concentration equals that at the blood inlet, then blood clearance equals the dialysate flow rate. In intermittent dialysis we attempt to achieve dialysate flow rates of twice the blood flow rate so that dialysate never approaches saturation. Saturated dialysate has no concentration gradient and leads to inefficient dialysis.

Convection

Convection is the movement of an array of species (ions, molecules, etc.) as a unit, driven in a specific direction and rate by an externally imposed force. Convective solute transport is the movement of solute that accompanies the movement of its solvent, in essence, the coupling of solute with its solvent as the solvent is driven through the semi-permeable membrane. The external driving force is the hydrostatic transmembrane pressure (TMP), which could be derived by physical (blood side positive pressure pump or filtrate side negative pressure pump) or chemical means (e.g. osmotic activity in dialysate). The hydrodynamic flow across the membrane is determined by the pressure difference, the surface area, and the intrinsic hydraulic permeability of the membrane in question. For CRRT that exploits convection, membranes are selected specifically for their high hydraulic permeability, also known as 'high flux.' Thus, there is a large bulk flow of plasma water and its dissolved constituents. Ultimately, the water channel pore size limits the flow of solutes that are large, such that in clinical practice, it is unlikely that there is appreciative convection of molecules larger than 20 kDa. Manufacturers test this property in aqueous solutions and claim higher molecular weight cutoffs, but *in vivo* operation in protein solutions markedly reduces the functional pore size because proteins and cells foul the membrane. The hydrostatic driving pressure jams the larger species up against the membrane and even into the pores. This can be a positive event if adsorption to the membrane is desired and this pressure utilizes all of the adsorptive surface area (see below). However, this membrane fouling limits the size of molecules being convectively transported. Nonetheless, the size of molecules transported convectively considerably exceeds that during diffusion. Thus, convection is the favored transport process if the goal is to remove middle or larger molecular weight species, such as mediators of sepsis.

The sieving coefficient is a measure of a solute's ability to convectively permeate a membrane. It is estimated by the ratio of the concentrations of the species in the filtrate divided by that in the plasma water (or blood, for ease of simplicity). A value of 1.0 demonstrates complete permeability and a value of zero reflects complete rejection. Molecular size plays a minor role in sieving up to approximately 8–12 kDa, then starts to affect convective transport more. Albumin (69 kDa) has a sieving coefficient of near zero, such that species bound to albumin will remain in the retentate. Albumin bound drugs are an example of the clinical relevance of this phenomenon. The clearance by convection is measured by the product of the filtration rate times the sieving coefficient. Thus, there is a linear relationship between clearance and the filtration rate, and the magnitude depends on the sieving coefficient. Most of the uremia related solutes have a sieving coefficient of unity and their clearance is the filtration rate.

Solute is removed via the bulk flow of plasma derived water with its dissolved constituents. As plasma water is driven across the membrane, retained constituents generate osmotic and oncotic forces to retard further filtration. A practical limit to filtration is ultimately reached. The driving force for the bulk flow is the TMP. Thus, maneuvers to increase solute removal will be directed towards increasing the filtration rate. This is achieved by increasing the TMP and by increasing the plasma water delivered to the membrane surface area. An extracorporeal blood pump achieves both of these goals concurrently.

Convection and diffusion can and do occur simultaneously. For all practical purposes clinically, these events occur independently and do not really affect each other. At extremes of clinical operating conditions, there may be interference, but this is not observed clinically.

Adsorption

Molecules adsorb to artificial membranes and this may represent a substantial removal from the circulation. Examples include several inflammatory cytokines adsorbing to AN69 and endotoxic peptides adsorbing to polysulfone. Convection enhances the efficiency of this by making more surface area available, essentially adding the surface area of the pores. By measuring a loss of mass from blood inlet to outlet and not observing that missing mass in the filtrate/dialysate, one infers that the mass has adsorbed to the membrane. Such adsorbed mass may in time be released off the membrane to end up back in the circulation or in the filtrate/dialysate. Nonetheless, adsorption represents a form of solute removal.

Concept of clearance

Solute clearance is defined as a volume of blood completely emptied of solute in a unit of time. It is an awkward and misleading concept, especially if the blood concentration of the solute is changing, as occurs during intermittent dialysis. Absolute solute removal is a much more meaningful measure, but has not been utilized because of the weight of history and experience with the concept of clearance. For CRRT where blood concentration of solute is relatively stable, the concept of clearance is far more useful. For example, if a steady state BUN concentration is 70 mg/dl, a clearance of 30 ml/min translates to the net removal of 2.1 mg/min. Performing CRRT for a day (1440 min) will lead to removal of 3024 mg of urea nitrogen. An intermittent HD treatment will remove two to three times this amount in an aggressive treatment. The clearance for the intermittent treatment may be seven times that for the CRRT, but the extended time performance of the CRRT makes up much of the clearance difference. CRRTs are probably equivalent to 4 to 5 intermittent treatments per week in total solute removal.

Application to CRRTs
CRRTs function for extended periods of time. Thus, a relatively low whole blood clearance (per minute) may reflect a substantial total removal

over the entire period. If the operating conditions are such that truly continuous operation is occurring, then clearances can be allowed to be lower. Since interruptions are not always predictable, it seems prudent to maximize blood flow, dialysate flow and filtration rates to the limit of practicality for each CRRT. Targets are a blood flow rate of 250 ml/min, and a dialysate or filtrate flow rate of 2 l/h or 34 ml/min.

4

The Prisma Machine

Ian Baldwin

The Prisma machine has been developed by Hospal (Lyon, France) specifically to perform the complete range of CRRT. Therefore, CVVH, SCUF, CVVHD, CVVHDF can all be performed with this machine.

This machine has several features which make it user friendly:

1. The control unit with 4 pumps (dialysate, blood, replacement fluid and effluent) with anticoagulant syringe and 3 weighing scales
2. Uses a disposable ready-to-connect set
3. Touch screen with smart built-in software that allows the performance of all desired operations. The screen provides step by step information to guide the nurse through circuit priming and operation
4. Monitoring of filter function by continuous measurement of pressure drop across the filter and of transmembrane pressure
5. Differential alarms to provide useful and timely information to assist the operator with trouble-shooting
6. Display of any fluid balance errors, air detection, blood leaks and altered pressures

The blood flow rate ranges from 10–180 ml/min, replacement flow rate between 0 and 2000 ml/h, dialysate rate from 0 to 2500 ml/h and effluent rate from 0 to 4500 ml/h.

The accuracy of fluid balance is ±0.45% at maximum flow rates. The pressure monitoring ranges are +50 mmHg to –250 mmHg for the arterial limb, –50 mmHg to +350 mmHg for the venous limb and –350 mmHg to +50 mmHg for the effluent line.

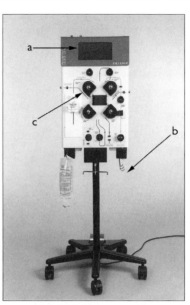

Figure 4.1: Front view of the Prisma CRRT machine. This machine has a number of distinguishing features, including: a) monochrome screen displaying operational functions, b) slimline body with stable five-wheel base stand, c) identical mini roller pumps in symmetrical layout.

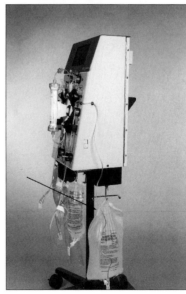

Figure 4.2: Side view of machine displaying dialysate replacement fluid bag and tubing.

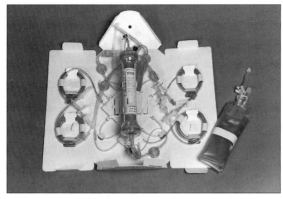

Figure 4.3: Integrated filter and tubing cartridge making set up easy. Each tubing coil corresponds to each roller pump for easy fit.

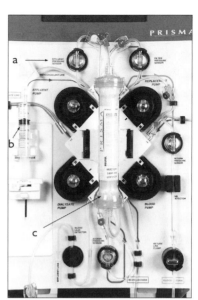

Figure 4.5: a) In-line pressure transducer pod within blood path, b) syringe driver for heparin infusion, c) filter with AN 69 membrane in operative position.

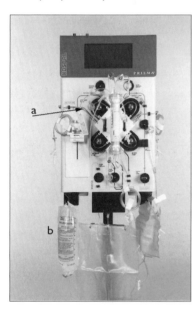

Figure 4.4: Close-up view of loaded circuit illustrating position of tubing for blood and dialysate pathways. a) Filter and tubing cartridge after loading onto machine, b) priming fluid and waste bag hanging on electronic scales.

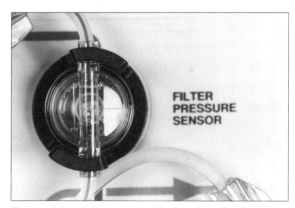

Figure 4.6: Close-up view of pressure pod locked in its holding bracket. Pressure obtained here is used to derive transmembrane pressure.

The anticoagulation set-up can deliver the anticoagulant by continuous infusion or as a bolus, with a range between 0 and 5 ml/hr.

6. Continuous recording of CRRT history for last 24 hours
7. First device solely developed for CRRT

Advantages
1. Very user friendly priming and set up
2. User friendly touch screen interface and instructions
3. Rapidity of setting up
4. Easy to understand alarms and trouble-shooting
5. Ability to perform all forms of CRRT

Limitations
1. Need for specific dedicated circuit
2. Specific dedicated circuit more expensive than standard set-ups
3. Standard filter area <1 m^2
4. Blood flow limited to only 180 ml/min
5. More sophisticated technology has increased cost of machine

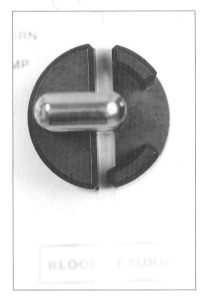

Figure 4.7:
Return blood line
clamp activated
by air detection.

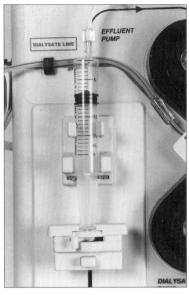

Figure 4.9:
Syringe driver for
the pre-filter
delivery of
anticoagulant.

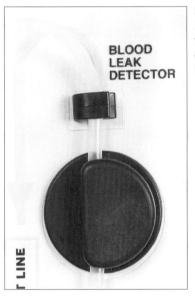

Figure 4.8:
Infrared system
for blood leak
detection
in effluent tubing.

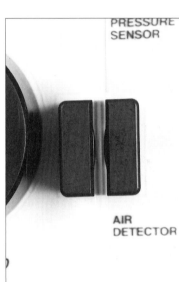

Figure 4.10:
Return blood
tubing passing
through
ultrasonic air
detecting device.

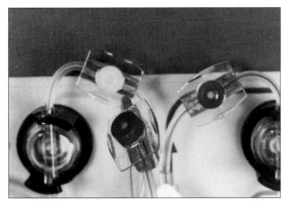

Figure 4.11: Close-up view of blood sampling ports. These ports can be used to remove air bubbles from the system.

5

The Baxter BM 25 machine

Ian Baldwin

The Baxter BM 25 (BM 11 & 14) machine

This machine consists of two integrated modules: the BM 11 (blood pump module) and the BM 14 (fluid delivery, removal and balancing module).

The blood module consists of a blood pump; air-in-line detector; blood leak detector; key pad and display field; two pressure transduction points and filter holder.

The blood pump delivers 350 ml/min and the pressure monitor for the outflow limb has a pressure range between –200 mmHg and +400 mmHg. The venous return pressure monitor operates between –50 mmHg and +350 mmHg.

The fluid balance monitor consists of a replacement fluid pump, an ultrafiltrate pump, an integrated weighing system for ultrafiltrate and replacement fluid, two pressure connection points (prefilter hydrostatic pressure and ultrafiltrate pressure), a fluids heater and an infusion stand.

The balance is controlled by scales with 1% accuracy. Each scale can carry up to 15 kg. The operational range for substitution fluid is between 100 ml and 9000 ml/h. The operational range for the ultrafiltration pump is between 100 ml and 11 000 ml/h. The net ultrafiltration rate can be set between 10 and 2000 ml/h. Control panels allow identification of changes in pressure. Installation of a dedicated tubing set permits operation in neonates and children. The heating system can warm up replacement fluid from 33 to 40°C. The machine can perform most blood purification treatments (CVVH, CVVHD, and plasma separation).

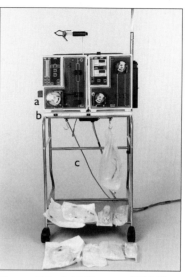

Figure 5.1: Initial layout of BM 25 machine. Circuit components assembled ready for priming procedure. Note, a) large roller pump for blood flow control, b) integrated double pump system for ultrafiltrate and replacement fluid control, and c) highly accurate weighing system to ensure accuracy of fluid balance.

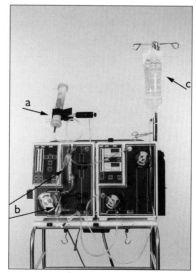

Figure 5.2: a) Hemofilter is now in place. Any membrane can be used in this system. b) Arterial component of blood circuit is now in place. c) Saline solution to allow priming of filter.

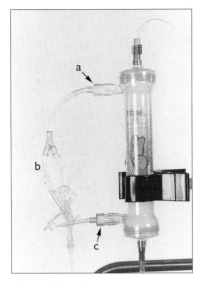

Figure 5.3: Close-up view of the hemofilter.
a) Note twin adapter connection to the ultrafiltrate port.
b) Sampling of ultrafiltrate is possible here.
c) Occlusive plug appropriate for CVVH mode. During CVVHD this port can be used for dialysate flow countercurrent to blood.

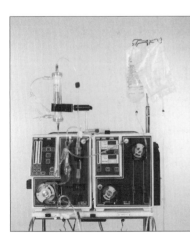

Figure 5.4: The venous line is now connected to out flow blood port of filter to complete the blood path of the circuit. Air detection is bypassed during this period to allow easy priming.

Advantages
1. Simple
2. Low cost
3. Any size filter can be used
4. High-volume CVVH can be performed due to ability of high blood flows and ultrafiltration rates
5. Disposables are reasonably priced
6. Good 'workhorse' in the ICU

Disadvantages
1. Limited 'diagnostics' available – no screen
2. More time-consuming priming procedure
3. Trouble-shooting somewhat laborious
4. Pressure displays of limited precision
5. Operating instructions to machine not intuitive
6. Heater system door-plate somewhat unreliable

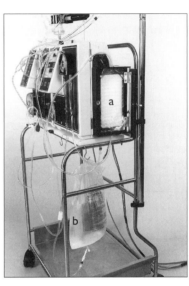

Figure 5.5:
a) The flat plate warming element allows warming of replacement or dialysis fluid depending on mode of therapy.
b) Replacement fluid hanging on scale is used for priming of replacement dialysate fluid path.

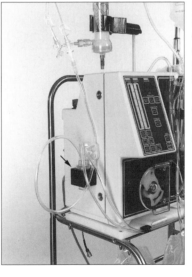

Figure 5.6:
Blood leak detector. This device detects presence of blood in the ultrafiltrate or dialysate, which indicates filter rupture.

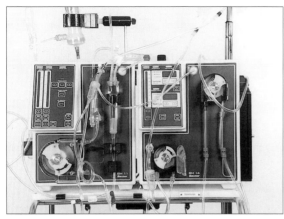

Figure 5.7: Completed circuit with blood and replacement fluid paths.

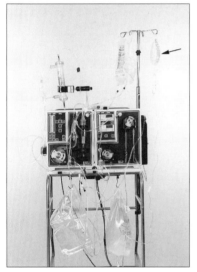

Figure 5.8: Complete picture of circuit indicating ultrafiltrate and replacement fluid bags for replacement fluid path and saline bag with arterial and venous spike connection for the blood path. A bag of normal saline (arrowed) is integrated into the circuit to simulate the patient with inflow and outflow.

A system/machine check should now be performed.

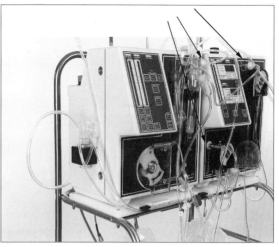

Figure 5.9: Close-up view of the circuit indicating the pressure transducers (arrowed) used for the monitoring of pre-filter pressure, post-filter (venous) pressure and ultrafiltrate pressure. The knowledge of such pressures permits the calculation of transmembrane pressure (TMP).

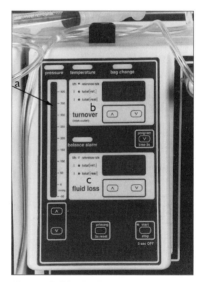

Figure 5.10: Push button control panel for ultrafiltration and replacement fluid. Also display for transmembrane pressure (a). The top panel (b) permits the planning and control of replacement fluid, ultrafiltration rate and total amount of fluid to be administered. The bottom panel (c) permits programming of ultrafiltration rate and total planned ultrafiltration fluid loss.

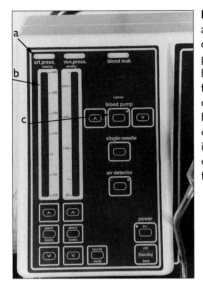

Figure 5.11:
a) Panel displaying pressure alarms. b) Alarm limits for pressure. c) Master blood pump control to increase or decrease blood flow rate.

6

The Gambro AK 10 (BMM 10/1) Machine

Ian Baldwin and Rinaldo Bellomo

The Gambro AK 10 Machine

This machine is basically derived from the blood module of the AK 10 produced by Gambro (Lund, Sweden) for the purpose of hemodialysis. It is most commonly used as a simple peristaltic blood pump with venous pressure display and safety features.

Blood flow rate can be set between 0 and 500 ml/min.

There is no display measurement of how much arterial pressure is applied to the outflow limb of the catheter to obtain the desired blood flow. An arterial line 'pillow' is decreased in size if excessive suction is applied and changes in size trigger the arterial pressure alarm. This pressure sensor is quite insensitive.

The venous return pressure is monitored by transducer and displayed continuously. A separate heparin pump is usually added and heparin delivered to the pre-filter position through a tubing attachment that is part of the circuit.

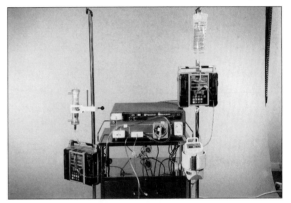

Figure 6.2: The filter and tubing circuit assembled on machine ready for priming with saline solution. The blood path tubing is initially primed with saline by gravity flow.

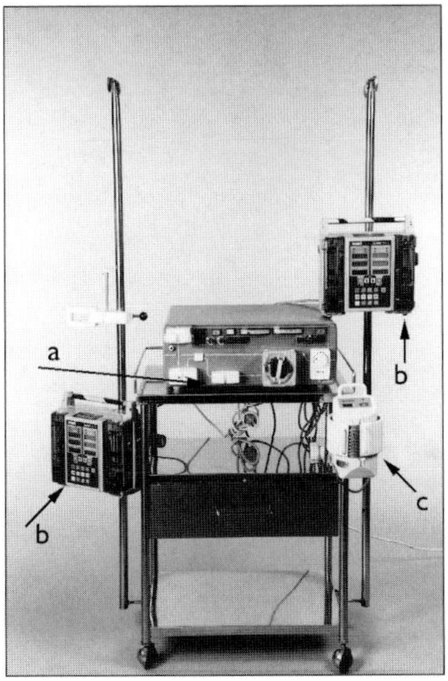

Figure 6.1: Gambro BMM 10/1 blood module with volumetric pumps for non-integrated pump-off hemofiltration system. a) Blood module on mobile console. b) Volumetric pumps for effluent and replacement fluid control. c) Replacement fluid warmer.

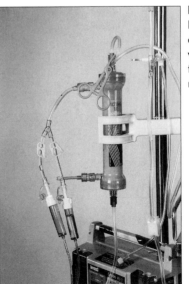

Figure 6.3A: Filter adapter for connection to IV volumetric pump for ultrafiltrate removal.

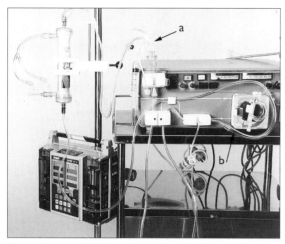

Figure 6.3B: a) Full blood path circuit in place with venous return line in position, b) peristaltic pump not yet in use to enable gravity dependent flow of saline solution.

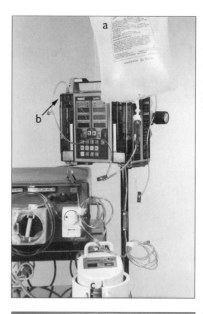

Figure 6.4: Replacement fluid (a) in position for delivery via IV pump (b) and warmer (c).

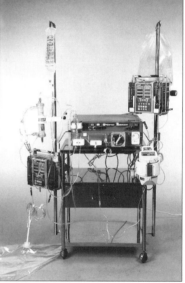

Figure 6.5: Complete circuit with blood path, replacement fluid and ultrafiltration pump-off and collection system.

This machine can be used to perform either CVVH or CVVHD or CVVHDF in a spontaneous ultrafiltration mode. The ultrafiltrate is then measured and replaced in part or in total as desired. This approach is labor intensive.

A preferred option is to use IV infusion (volumetric) pumps to control ultrafiltration and replacement fluid or dialysate flow. Such pumps are widely available in any ICU and can be connected to the circuit via appropriate tubing. In CVVH, for instance, the desired ultrafiltrate flow rate can then be set at 1, 1.5 or 2 l/h. The replacement fluid is then set as desired. If volume loss is planned for, the replacement fluid rate will be ≥100–200 ml short of the ultrafiltration rate. If no fluid loss is desired, the replacement fluid rate is the same as the ultrafiltration rate.

All of these pumps, however, are a makeshift combination of various pieces, which were separately produced or intended to be self-standing. The integration of these pumps is not always satisfactory. Continued filtration by volumetric pumps can occur while the blood flow has stopped due to access problems. This phenomenon is due to lack of integration between the two systems that will lead to filter clotting. Furthermore, volumetric pumps are inaccurate by ± 3–5% of infused volume. This means that if CVVH is performed at 2 l/h (48 l/day), there could be an error of 2–3 l in fluid balance (i.e. the set fluid balance is not the

real fluid balance). Despite these shortcomings this makeshift system is satisfactory in most cases, is flexible and is very cheap compared with other solutions to the problem of giving CRRT. It is particularly useful in developing countries where the money may not be available to buy machines that are more sophisticated and purpose built.

Advantages
1. Cheap (approximate cost for blood module: US$ 2000 – volumetric pumps usually already available in the ICU. Their cost is about

US$ 2000 for a set of two for a total approximate system cost of US$ 4000).
2. Simple technology
3. Easy to learn and intuitive set up
4. Flexible
5. Disposables are also flexible and cheap
6. Can perform any CRRT therapy and plasmapheresis as well if appropriate filter is used

Disadvantages

1. Makeshift arrangement
2. Inaccurate fluid balance all the time and very inaccurate fluid balance if transmembrane pressure is high with potential risk to patient
3. Inaccurate blood pump
4. Full set-up takes up to 1 hour
5. No monitoring of transmembrane pressure
6. Insensitive alarms, particularly outflow–arterial

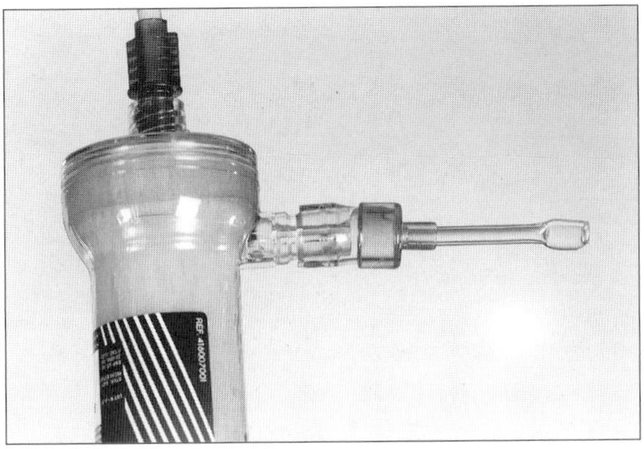

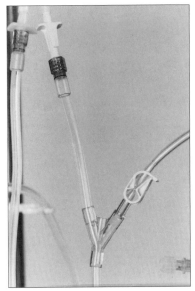

Figure 6.6B: Y connection in 'arterial' limb of circuit. This connection allows administration of flush solution to return blood from circuit to patient. Arterial limb if clamped off to do this.

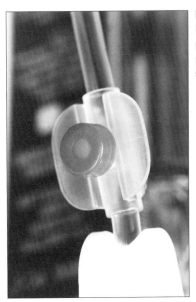

Figure 6.6C: Blood sampling port for pre- and post-filter blood sampling.

Figure 6.6A: Occlusion of second filter port. This occlusion is necessary during CVVH. In CVVHD this port is used for dialysate outflow.

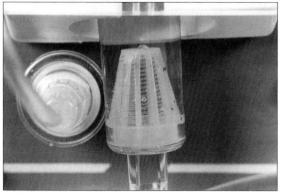

Figure 6.6D: Filter at bottom of bubble trap to prevent large clot from returning to patient.

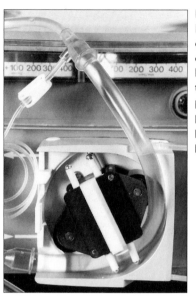

Figure 6.7: Blood pump cassette with compressible large diameter tubing (adult patient) being placed in correct position after priming.

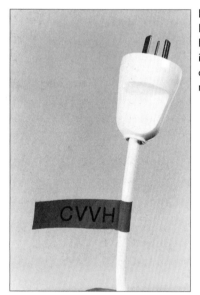

Figure 6.6E: Master plug labelled for easy identification in case of malfunction.

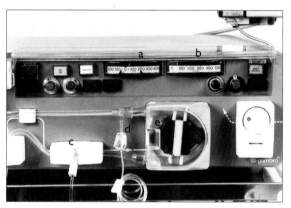

Figure 6.8: a) venous pressure display, b) Pump speed display, c) arterial pressure sensing plate, d) heparin line, e) peristaltic pump and tubing ready for function.

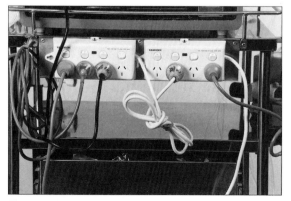

Figure 6.6F: Multiplug electrical adapter needed to supply power to module, warmer and IV pumps.

7.

The Hygieia 'Plus' Machine

Ian Baldwin and Rinaldo Bellomo

The Hygieia 'Plus' CRRT Machine

This is a custom made machine for continuous therapies. The machine incorporates many features of a conventional dialysis circuit with modification for CRRT. The circuit tubing is created with separate components for the 'outflow' and 'return' blood lines, fluids replacement and removal lines. Pressure sensor lines are formed into the tubing to determine pre/post membrane and TMP (UF line) readings. An air trap chamber and blood leak detector make this circuit 'conventional' and easily understand for those experienced with dialysis equipment. The new feature of this circuit is the replacement fluids and ultrafiltrate removal measurement system which uses large collection chambers to measure fluids accurately by infra-red detectors. Roller pumps control the fluids to manage set replacement and removal rates.

The main machine unit sits on top of a trolley cabinet making a suitable machine working height for most staff. The circuit fits to the front and both sides of the machine (3 separate areas) distinguishing blood–membrane path from fluids management.

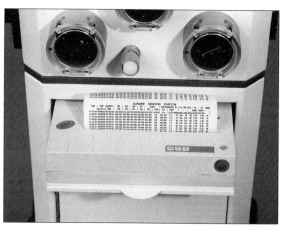

Figure 7.1B: Vertical arrangement incorporates a printer and storage cabinet below this.

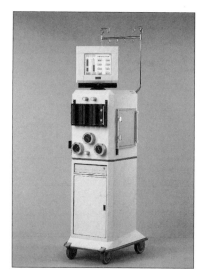

Figure 7.2A: This side of the machine has a large surface area fluids warming plate adjacent to fluid chamber holders.

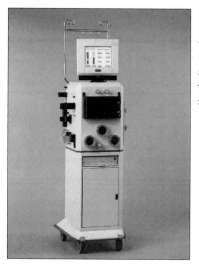

Figure 7.1A: Hygieia Plus CRRT machine integrates blood and fluid pumps via a color touch screen.

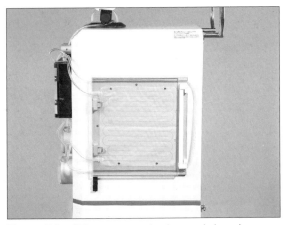

Figure 7.2B: Tubing cassette in place and clear door closes to insulate but maintain visibility.

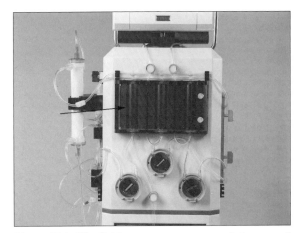

Figure 7.4: The fluids management system is integrated into the touch screen control above. Infra-red measurement of all fluids is via 100 ml plastic chambers in a holder (arrowed).

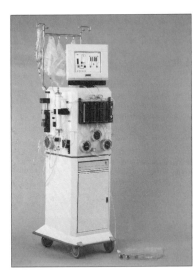

Figure 7.3: Hygiea Plus ready for treatment with conventional disposables circuit and filter. The blood path is on the side of the machine and the fluids management is on the front.

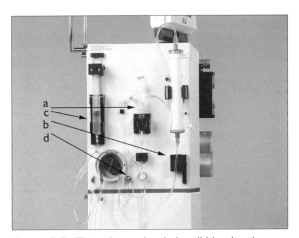

Figure 7.5: This side panel includes all blood path tubing and filter with conventional design: a) venous air trap chamber, b) air and blood leak detection sensors, c) anticoagulant syringe driver. Pressure sensors are incorporated to determine venous resistance and TMP (d).

The color user interface screen for machine and technique control is touch sensitive and has several different configurations. It can be an 'animation' of the treatment in use, or display data for settings and real time circuit monitoring/fluid balance. Anticoagulation can be incorporated into the circuit via an optional syringe driver or separate IV pump.

Priming and initiation of treatment is achieved by on screen prompts and sequential instructions making this machine good for teaching and self-direction. A log of treatment history and suggestions to remedy alarm functions are helpful and diagnostic of impending failure or incorrect fluid balance.

This machine appears to have many good features and should prove to be popular in the continuous therapies setting in ICU.

Advantages

1. Conventional circuit enabling changes to separate sections of the tubing circuit. e.g. venous line.

2. The height and presentation of the machine at the bedside make it ergonomically suitable for nurses.
3. The heater–fluids warmer is of a large surface area and offers low resistance to fluids flow.
4. Touch screen interaction with priming and troubleshooting prompts is helpful for learning and teaching use of this machine.
5. Fluids management is by infra-red sensors and potentially very accurate eliminating the use of scales to weigh fluids hanging under the machine. Fluid waste can be direct to discharge with this machine.

Disadvantages

1. Pressure sensing lines may be prone to clotting with blood and then becoming inaccurate.
2. Replacement fluids bags are required to hang above the machine on a bar–hook which can be at a difficult height to lift to for some nurses.
3. The venous air chamber may be a point for clot development as for all circuits designed this way.
4. The machine is competitive on costing but may be prohibitive for some.

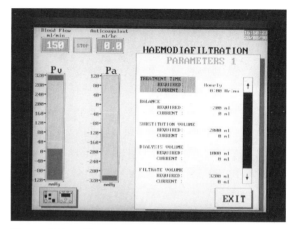

Figure 7.6B: Alarm displays for blood path.

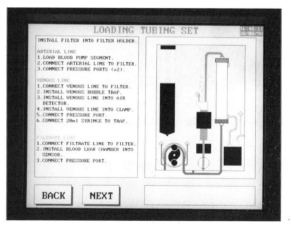

Figure 7.7: The fitting of the tubing circuit is demonstrated and described on this screen to direct, sequential priming procedure. This is assisted by color-coding.

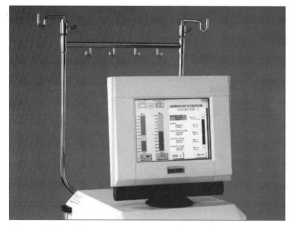

Figure 7.6A: Parameters screen allows all treatment parameters to be set and controlled. The replacement and/or dialysate fluids holder bar can be seen behind this screen.

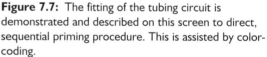
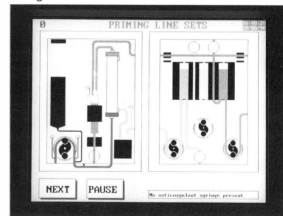

Figure 7.8: Animation display indicates real-time progress during priming sequence. There is a touch roller pump icon to facilitate priming when prompted.

8

The Diapact CRRT Machine

Lynne Snyder for B. Braun Medical Inc.

The Diapact CRRT Machine

The last generation Diapact CRRT machine by B. Braun is a compact self-contained system for all types of CRRT treatment including high-volume therapy. This machine follows a series of previous models and has been developed to meet all CRRT needs.

The new machine has a simplified operating interface and built-in software to assist the operator with priming and conduct of therapy. It has a high resolution screen for optimal readability. Alarms operate acoustically and optically with a clear description of the cause to assist in trouble-shooting.

The Diapact machine allows the operator to perform all types of CRRT and plasma treatment therapies. The system uses 3 pumps. The blood pump operates in a range between 20 and 300 ml/min, while the dialysate/ultrafiltrate outflow and the dialysate/replacement fluid inflow pumps also operate with a range that reaches 300 ml/min.

Fluid balance is achieved with an accurate weighing system, which can hold up to 25 l. An effective fluid warming cell allows the administration of high-flow, prewarmed fluids.

Dialysate can be recirculated to achieve equilibrium with plasma (filtration/backfiltration) through a mechanism combining convection and diffusion (continuous high-flux dialysis).

Advantages
1. Flexible
2. Can perform all therapies
3. Can perform continuous high-flux dialysis with recirculation of dialysate
4. Decreased waste generation
5. Can perform high volume therapies
6. User friendly visual display
7. User friendly alarm system

Disdvantages
1. Somewhat bulky
2. Pre-assembled tubing kit exclusive for this machine

Table 8.1: Detailed display of functions for the three different pumps

Kind of treatment	Pump no. 1	Pump no. 2	Pump no. 3	Kind of filter	Kind of solution
CVVH/HF Double needle	AP	UFP	IP	HF	Bic./lact. buffer
HF (IVVH) Single needle	AP	VP	IP	HF	Bic. buffer
CVVHD/HD Double needle	AP	UFP	DP	LF	Bic. buffer
CVVHFD/HFD Double needle	AP	UFP	DP	HF	Bic./lact. buffer
CVVHFD/HFD Single needle	AP	VP	DP	HF	Bic./lact. buffer

AP = Arterial Pump, VP = Venous Pump, UFP = Ultrafiltration Pump, IP = Infusion Pump, DP = Dialysate Pump.

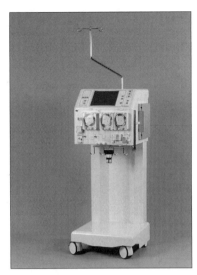

Figure 8.1: Full view of Diapact machine. Please note unique three-pump system, wide color screen and side fluid warmer.

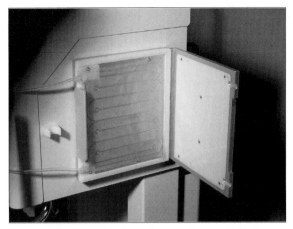

Figure 8.3: Close-up view of the replacement fluid warmer, which works as a plate warmer system.

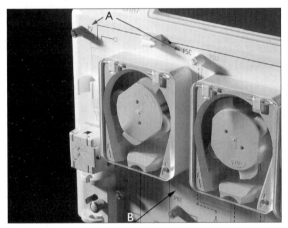

Figure 8.2: Close up view of blood flow and UF flow pumps and pressure sensors. Arrows marked (A) display the site of connection for return venous pressure (left) and the connection for switching chamber pressure measurement in single needle mode or for fluid outlet pressure measurement. The arrow marked (B) indicates the pressure sensor for pre-filter pressure measurement.

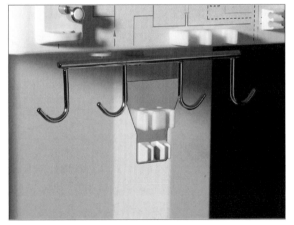

Figure 8.4: Close-up view of the hanging and weighing system for the dialysate or replacement fluid and ultrafiltrate. Just above that, one can see the circuit lines designed on to the machine front to facilitate the positioning of the tubing.

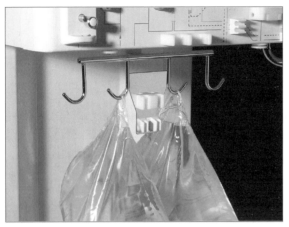

Figure 8.5: Weighing system with ultrafiltrate and replacement fluid bags in position. Just above that, one can see the plastic prefilter and switching chambers holder.

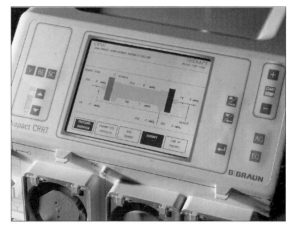

Figure 8.7: Graphic display of the circuit in CVVH mode with information on circuit pressure and the ability to control circuit settings.

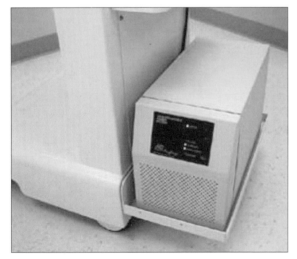

Figure 8.6: Optional internal battery pack, which allows the performance of treatments for some hours when the main power supply fails.

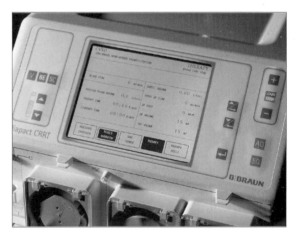

Figure 8.8: Graphic display of command functions during CVVH, which allows the nurse to set parameters as well as provide information on areas of circuit dysfunction.

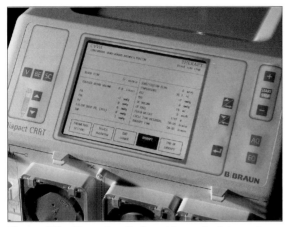

Figure 8.9: Operative display with recall of data using the 'History' button, which allows the operator to obtain information on the details of the therapy from the time the new circuit was set up.

9

The EQUAsmart Machine

Luciano Fecondini for Medica Pty Ltd *with Flaviano Ghiotto*

This device is produced by Medica (Medolla, Modena, Italy) and is the result of a continuing evolution of the EQUA line of CRRT machines into more sophisticated devices.

This integrated CRRT system can deliver SCUF, CVVH and CVVHDF treatment. It has many interesting features. The fluid load cell is at an ideal height for easy access. The filter holder can function for neonatal and adult therapies. An anticoagulant delivery syringe is incorporated. This machine uses a two-pump system: one pump for blood flow and the other for the delivery of replacement fluid. There is no pump control of ultrafiltration, which is allowed to proceed spontaneously. The ultrafiltrate is continuously weighed and the information derived, together with the planned fluid loss entered into the software of the machine by the nurse or physician, is used to regulate the fluid replacement pump rate. The rate of spontaneous ultrafiltration will depend on blood flow and filter condition. This choice to abandon pump-off technology is aimed at prolonging filter life. Correct fluid replacement is ensured by the presence of three highly accurate balancing systems (ultrafiltrate, replacement fluid and dialysate).

The machine contains standard safety features (warmer, blood leak detector, air leak detector, monitoring of arterial, venous and ultrafiltrate pressure). The instructions for priming are easy to follow. The display of treatment instruction, treatment setting and current operating conditions is comprehensive, user friendly and visually appealing.

Another interesting and useful feature is the ability to print information on the operation of the filter over a given period of time.

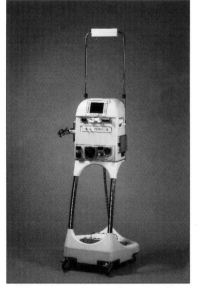

Figure 9.1: EQUAsmart is an integrated system intended for use in intensive care units for critically ill patients with acute renal failure (ARF) being treated with slow continuous ultrafiltration (SCUF), continuous veno-venous hemofiltration (CVVH) and continuous veno-venous hemodiafiltration (CVVHDF).

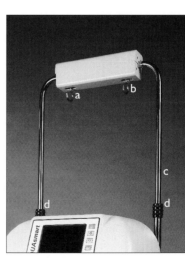

Figure 9.2: The upper part of the EQUAsmart machine.
a) Dialysate load cell,
b) replacement solution load cell,
c) up/down sliding holder,
d) tightening knobs for holder.

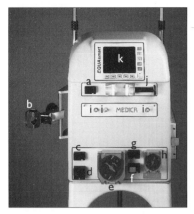

Figure 9.3: Front view. a) Adjustment clamp for dialysate in. b) Filter holder designed for neonatal, pediatric and adult filters. c) Adjustment clamp for ultrafiltrate/effluent line. d) Blood leak detector on ultrafiltrate/effluent line. e) Blood pump; flow rate is programmable from 10–400 ml/min. f) Safety clamp on venous line. g) Air detector on venous line. h) Replacement solution pump: flow rate is balance managed from 0–150 ml/min. i) Three pressure measurement ports: arterial, filter (pressure drop) and venous. j) Anticoagulant syringe pump: programmable in bolus or continuous mode. k) Control panel with color graphic display and active user interface.

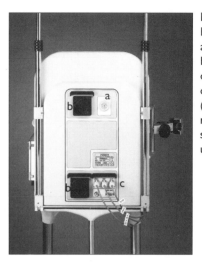

Figure 9.5: Rear view. a) Audible alarm. b) Cooling fans. c) Load cell connectors (dialysate, replacement solution and ultrafiltrate).

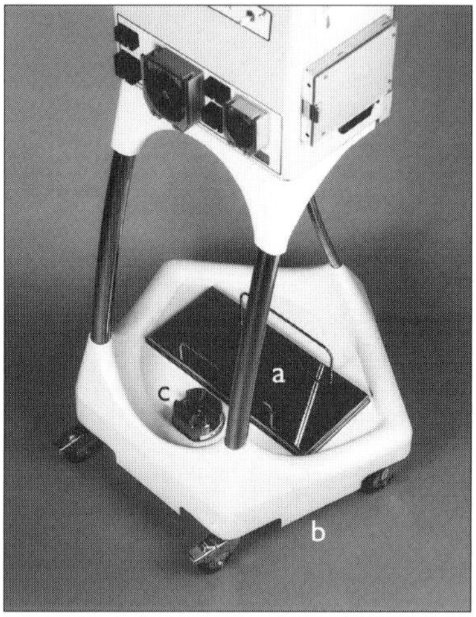

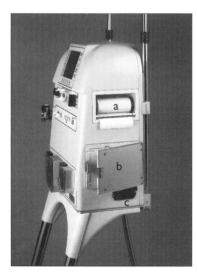

Figure 9.4: Side view. a) Printer for treatment data. b) Flat plate warmer for warming bag. c) Power supply assembly.

Figure 9.6: The lower part of the EQUAsmart machine. a) Ultrafiltrate load cell. b) Five wheels for easy transportation: two of them can be locked for safe operation. c) 2 kg calibration weight for load cells.

Advantages
1. Excellent visual display.
2. Only two pumps with associated circuit simplicity.
3. Anticoagulant delivery system.
4. Comprehensive monitoring.
5. Accurate weighing system.
6. Built for neonatal and adult use.
7. Easy set-up.
8. Cost.

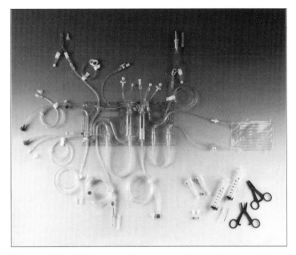

Figure 9.7: Tubing set: A compact disposable cartridge that includes all the tubings has been developed for easy patient connection and treatment start-up. The cartridge has a low priming volume and gives the physician and nursing staff the flexibility of choice of pre-dilution and post-dilution treatments.

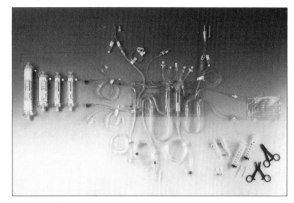

Figure 9.8: Tubing set and hemofilters/hemodiafilters: This compact disposable cartridge has been developed in order to leave the physician the choice of the most suitable filter for the patient treatment (neonatal, pediatric or adult).

Disadvantages

1. Because of lack of pump-off system, unable to perform pure CVVHD.
2. High-volume therapy only possible if large filter in use with limited loss of filtering surface.
3. If large filter used, spontaneous ultrafiltration may exceed replacement fluid specifications (unlikely event) requiring the nurse to decrease blood flow.
4. Custom-made manufacturer's tubing necessary.
5. Somewhat vertically bulky.

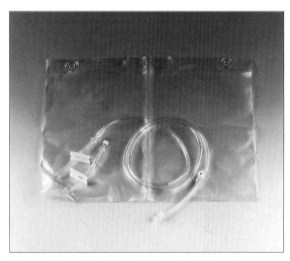

Figure 9.9A: Ultrafiltrate/effluent bag (7 litres).

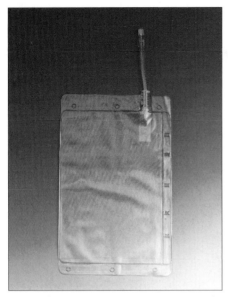

Figure 9.9B: Drainage bag for priming with non-return valve (2 litres).

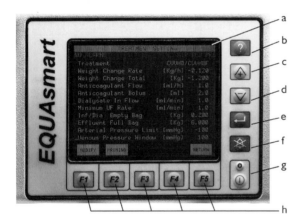

Figure 9.10: The control panel in treatment setting mode. a) graphic color display. b) help in line key. c) increasing value/up selection key. d) decreasing value/down selection key. e) enter/confirmation key. f) mute alarm key. g) on/off switch. h) function keys: each relevant function is displayed in the nearby area of the display.

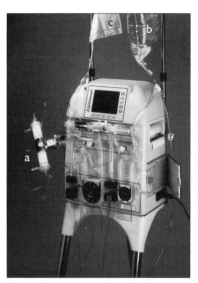

Figure 9.11: The machine is ready for priming. a) Hemofilter/hemodiafilter, b) the priming solution bag on the replacement solution load cell, c) 2 l drainage bag on the dialysate load cell.

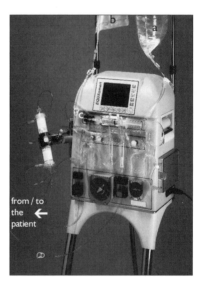

Figure 9.12: SCUF and CVVH treatment. a) Replacement solution bag, b) 2 l drainage bag, c) during SCUF or CVVH treatment the adjustable clamp for dialysate-in is normally closed.

from / to the patient ←

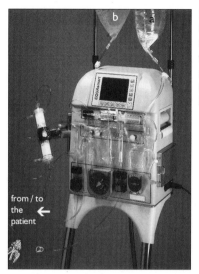

Figure 9.13: CVVHD/ CVVHDF treatment. a) Replacement solution bag, b) dialysate bag.

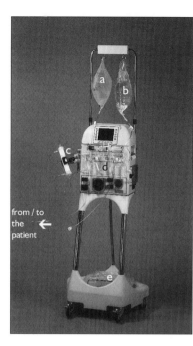

Figure 9.15: EQUAsmart during treatments. a) Dialysate bag (not present in SCUF/CVVH treatments), b) replacement solution bag, c) hemofilter/ hemodiafilter, d) disposable cartidge, e) ultrafiltrate/ effluent bag.

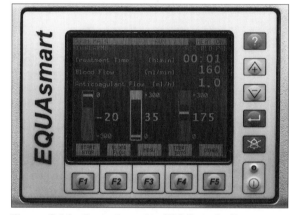

Figure 9.14: Control panel in 'RUN' mode. During treatment, the basic conditions are displayed in the main screen of running mode: other information about treatment is available in other screens.

10.

The Multimat B IC Machine

Ciro Tetta for Bellco Pty Ltd *with Flaviano Ghiotto*

This machine is manufactured by Bellco S.p.a. (Mirandola, Modena, Italy). This device is derived from an intermittent dialysis machine and is characterized by an easy interface and linear screen, which provide for a self-learning preparation and installation of the circuit. The circuit is color-coded for easy identification of components. The machine uses a double pump system, which controls ultrafiltration and reinfusion (or dialysate in and out in dialysis mode) and, of course, blood flow. During CVVH, one pump (equipped with a double tubing set) serves as the controller for blood flow and reinfusion fluid at a proportion of 100 to 15, with maximal values of 400 and 60 ml/min respectively. This approach ensures that the filtration fraction is always maintained at less than 20%, thus minimizing hemoconcentration and potentially maximizing filter life. In the CVVHD

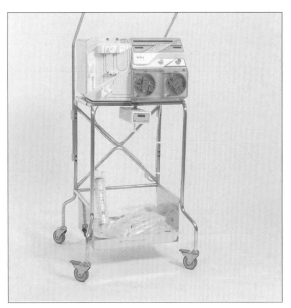

Figure 10.2: The trolley allows easy transportation of both the module and the disposables necessary for treatment.

or CVVHDF mode, the blood flow to dialysate flow proportion is 100 to 30 resulting in a maximum dialysate delivery rate of 120 ml/min. This proportional system ensures that there is optimal equilibration between blood and dialysate urea concentration. Thus little dialysate is wasted, while maximal urea clearance is achieved for a given dialysate delivery. The proportioning system is achieved by the use of tubing of different internal diameters. A fluid balancing system ensures the accuracy of the volumetric control created by the pumps. The machine is easily transportable and has standard safety features: blood detector in the ultrafiltrate line, air detector in the infusion line, arterial and venous pressure detector, pre-filter pressure detector and the obvious connection between the blood flow and ultrafiltrate flow pump (same pump) ensuring that when blood flow stops, ultrafiltration also stops.

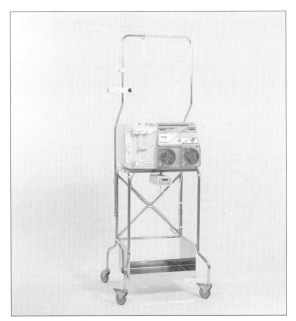

Figure 10.1: The double pump architecture Multimat B IC performs most common therapies, such as: SCUF, CVVH, CVVHD.

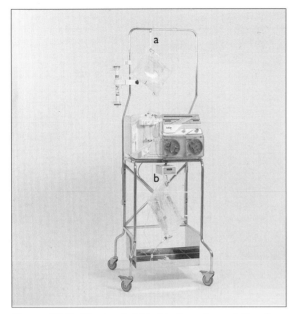

Figure 10.3: The hook (a) holds the saline solution for the priming procedure. The scale (b) ensures real-time monitoring of the fluid balance for both replacement and ultrafiltrate collecting bags (up to 20 kg).

Advantages

1. Simple preparation and monitoring.
2. Capacity to handle fluids of up to 25 kg in weighing system.
3. Accuracy of weighing system.
4. Proportional blood flow/ultrafiltrate system ensuring safe filtration fraction.
5. Proportional blood flow/dialysate system ensuring efficient utilization of dialysate.
6. Stable trolley which occupies limited space.
7. Ability to use different filters.
8. Cost.

Disadvantages

1. Screen is small and sometimes difficult to read.
2. Need for special custom-made manufacturer's tubing to perform therapy.
3. Need to use different tubing sets for CVVH and CVVHD.
4. Heparin pump is not incorporated.
5. Limitations on ultrafiltration fraction make high-volume convective therapy (high-volume CVVH) impossible.
6. No display of delta weight on scale requiring screen check.

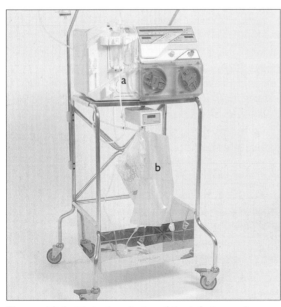

Figure 10.4: Note the placing of the infusion and ultrafiltration lines (a) and the replacement ultrafiltrate-collecting bags on the scale (b). Also note the placing of the arterial and venous lines.

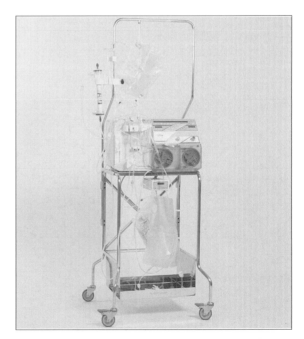

Figure 10.5: The machine is now ready to start the priming procedure.

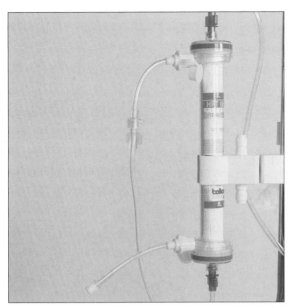

Figure 10.6: Note the filter adapters, which allow safe connection to any kind of dializer.

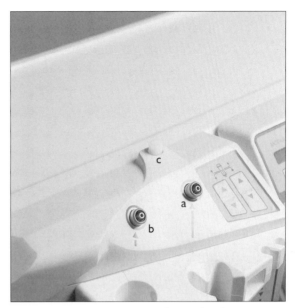

Figure 10.8: The Multimat B IC provides three pressure detections; a) arterial pressure, b) venous pressure, c) blood prefilter pressure.

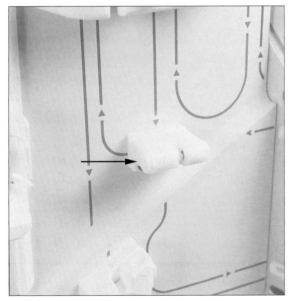

Figure 10.7: The blood leak detector (BLD), arrowed, placed on the ultrafiltrate line ensures control of the filter integrity. If a BLD alarm occurs the machine will immediately alert the operator.

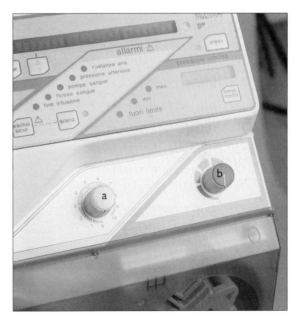

Figure 10.9: Note the knobs which adjust ultrafiltration rate and a) Qb/Qinf (in CVVH), and b) Qb/Qd (in CVVHD).

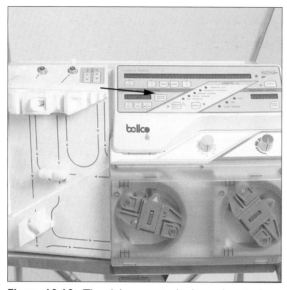

Figure 10.10: The alphanumeric display and control panel (arrowed) allows all the adjustments and operating parameters and alarms visualization.

11

The Aquarius Machine

Gerhard Marquart and Meg Blogg for Edwards life sciences Pty Ltd

The Aquarius is an integrated unit that can perform all types of blood purification therapies (CVVH, CVVHD, CVVHDF, SCUF and plasmafiltration).

The module contains four roller pumps that are color coded. The blood pump (red) delivers up to 450 ml/min. Pump inflow and outflow pressures are monitored and the values displayed. The arterial outflow access pressure (pre-pump) range is − 300–200 mmHg, whilst the venous return pressure (post pump) range is −50–350 mmHg. Pressure domes snap into position and have no blood–air interface. There is an ultrasonic air detector beneath the venous chamber, which controls the line clamp to prevent air embolism.

Fluid exchange is controlled by a balancing weigh scale, which allows delivery of up to 10 l/h and net fluid removal of 3 l/h. The fluid delivery/removal system operates by means of three roller pumps with an accuracy of ±1%. The post dilution pump (green) is the control pump and ensures balance accuracy by regulating its function every second.

The predilution (blue) roller pump delivers solution at a fixed rate, either as substitution solution or as dialysate. With CVVHD, when only one pump is used, the scale regulates this pump. Pre- and postdilution may be shared during therapy and rates may be adjusted at any time. The filtrate pump (yellow) removes up to 13 l/h with a net fluid removal of 0–3000 ml/h. An efficient coil tubing design allows heating up to 39°C of replacement solution of up to 6 l/h. This enables high volume exchanges without significant thermal loss.

The Aquarius has an interactive TFT color screen. A single selector knob guides all functions. The screen displays the modes of operation, flow rates, pressures, treatment parameters, alarms and includes instructional schematics. The screen can be swivelled 360° to enable viewing from any angle.

The Aquarius unit has both audible and visual alarms. There is a printing capacity and a PCMA card, which is optional.

All therapy types are set up with the same set of lines. The tubing for blood and solution lines comes as a single moulded tubing set, which is color coded for ease of insertion, identification and priming. Priming is automated with auto-loading and with the ability to hang the priming bags on the side of the machine. There is no pre-set filter size requirement, so that filters of different size and membranes can be used for therapy.

Advantages
1. Incorporated syringe driver for heparin anticoagulation
2. High volume hemofiltration
3. Automated priming
4. Filter flexibility
5. All therapy types
6. Minimal blood–air interface
7. 10.4 inch (26 cm) color TFT screen
8. Efficient fluid warmer
9. One set for all therapies
10. Therapy parameters can be changed at any time

Disadvantages
1. Citrate anticoagulation capacity not yet developed
2. New design without clinical history
3. Unable to pre-dilute with CVVHDF
4. May be heavy to transport at 75 kg

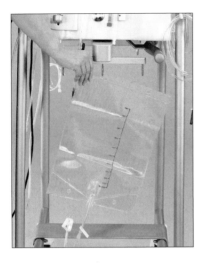

Figure 11.1: Aquarius machine ready for operation

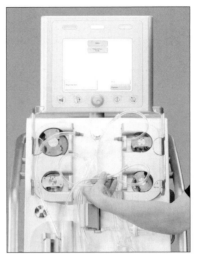

Figure 11.3: The blood and solution lines are a single molded tubing set, color coded for simple set up. The one set is used for all therapy types. In preparation mode the tubing is auto loaded onto the roller pumps. Roller pumps are color-coded:
Red   – larger roller pump for blood
Yellow   – ultrafiltrate
Green   – postdilution
Blue   – predilution/dialysate
Any filter can be used. A graded filter holder allows the use of pediatric and neonatal filters. Connection of lines to the filter makes set up complete.

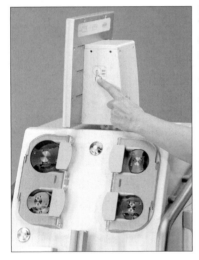

Figure 11.2: The On/Off switch is on the right side of the monitor screen. This is operational when the mains power is switched on.

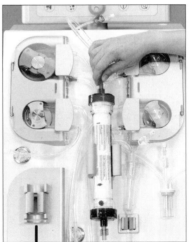

Figure 11.4: Pressure domes snap into position. There is no air interface to monitor pressures.

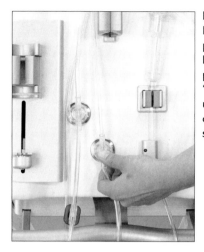

Figure 11.5: Pre- and/or postdilution may be selected. The predilution line is 'free' and may be used for dialysate or predilution substitution.

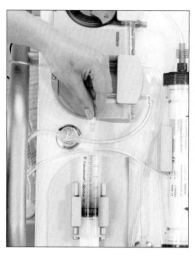

Figure 11.8: Ultrafiltrate collection bags are hung on the balancing weigh scale. The weigh scale pulls out for easy placement and removal of bags (20 kg maximum).

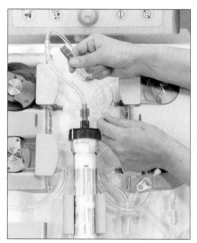

Figure 11.6: Sitting beneath the venous return chamber the ultrasonic air detector is unlikely to pick up artifact from turbulence in the venous return chamber.

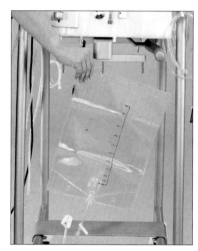

Figure 11.9: Substitution and/or dialysate solution is hung opposite the ultrafiltrate bags. Weigh scale accuracy is ±1° and regulated every second (20 kg maximum).

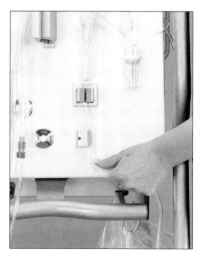

Figure 11.7: Any 30 ml or 50 ml syringe may be used for heparin anticoagulation. There is a 1 ml bolus function. The delivery range is 0.5–15 ml/h. The heparin line included in the tubing set is connected to the syringe.

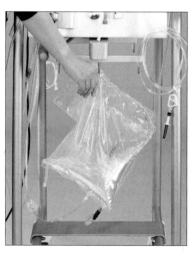

Figure 11.10: The fluid hangs compactly beneath the main body of the machine.

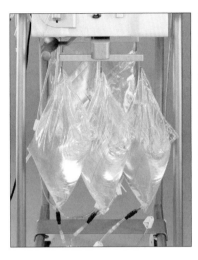

Figure 11.11:
A prime collection bag is included in the set up kit. Priming solution and collection bag are hung on the side of the machine; no IV pole is needed.

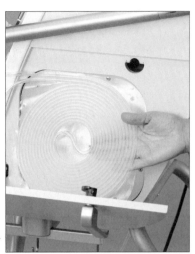

Figure 11.13:
Display screen with control panel in CVVH mode. Note prompts and operator query response system.

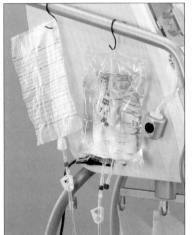

Figure 11.12:
A flat plate fluid warmer on the side of the machine houses the heating coil. Solution is warmed to 37°C up to 6 l/h. Temperature range is 35–39°C.

12

The RanD Performer Machine

Corrado Bellini for RanD S r l

The Performer machine is an integrated system that is able to support a variety of therapeutic applications in different medical fields (oncology, apheresis and dialysis), based on the principles of extracorporeal blood/fluid circulation, including the following CRRT techniques: SCUF, CVVH, CVVHD and CVVHDF.

As a result of its hardware and software platform, developed according to current state-of-the-art electronic technology and the principles of continuous dialytic techniques, the Performer machine is characterized by high performance, flexibility and user friendliness.

The main system features with reference to CRRT techniques are as follows:

Four self-occluding peristaltic pumps. These pumps have adjustable flow rates (20–500 ml/min for blood and 5–200 ml/min for solutions) according to the method in use; this feature allows performance of CVVH therapies with simultaneous and continuous pre-post filter infusion or CVVHDF therapies with independent post-filter infusion.

Monitoring of all important pressures detectable on the extracorporeal circuit both on the blood side and fluid side, for constant control of filter efficiency and patients' safety.

Patients' fluid balance control by means of overall monitoring (one single-load cell) of 'in–out' volumes; this configuration does not provide accurate values of specific exchange volumes but drastically reduces absolute error on overall volume (difference between volume in and volume out).

The system scales can be loaded with up to 20 l of solution (dialysate or replacement fluid) per single session for the selected therapy, with the possibility of replacement during the same therapy without interruption and/or parameter modification.

High-performance heater, which achieves adequate heating of the infusion solution even during high flow techniques.

Integrated syringe pump for anticoagulant administration, both continuous and discontinuous, to be used with 20 ml and 30 ml syringes.

Optional device for hematocrit and oxygen saturation (SAT-O_2) in-line measuring and monitoring, which can provide additional and important physiological information on volume status and overall physiological stability during CRRT.

Full-graphic (SVGA: 800×600, 256 colors) and 'user-friendly' operator interface, with 'touch screen' monitor. All symbols and operative functions are represented by self-explanatory icons. Moreover, all therapies (including all phases and subphases) are represented by dynamic flow diagrams for an easy and quick identification of the parameters status.

Optional integrated in-line printer (thermal printer, up to 102 digits/line) for real-time printouts of the current treatment main data.

Possibility of transferring data to an external PC through a serial port (RS485–232) with all data recorded during last treatment being retained until a new therapy is set up.

UPS (Uninterruptible Power Supply) with at least 30 min autonomy (heater excluded), particularly useful to carry on therapy in the event of blackouts.

Compact dimensions (total height can be reduced to 900 mm) for easy transportation and to facilitate transfers between clinical environments.

Advantages

1. Ability to perform all therapies with any filter/dialyzer
2. Ability to achieve high blood flows and ultrafiltrate flows necessary for high-volume hemofiltration treatment

3. State-of-the art electronics
4. Excellent user-friendly touch screen with color display to regulate and monitor therapy
5. Option for data printing and data downloading
6. Option to have in-line monitoring of hematocrit and oxygen saturation

Disadvantages

1. Can load only 20 l at a time, which may be a small practical shortcoming in high-volume therapies
2. Limited accuracy for total volumes exchanged (high accuracy for fluid balance)
3. Limited experience with the device outside of Europe

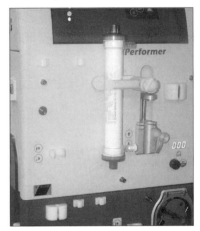

Figure 12.3: Blood circuit set-up: filter. For 'CRRT' therapies, the system is able to support different type of filters (low and high permeability) in a range from 0.5 to 2.0 sq. meter. The following steps describe the set-up of CVVH therapy mode.

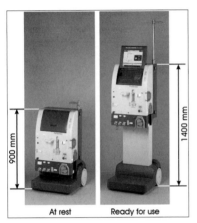

Figure 12.1: Equipment overview.

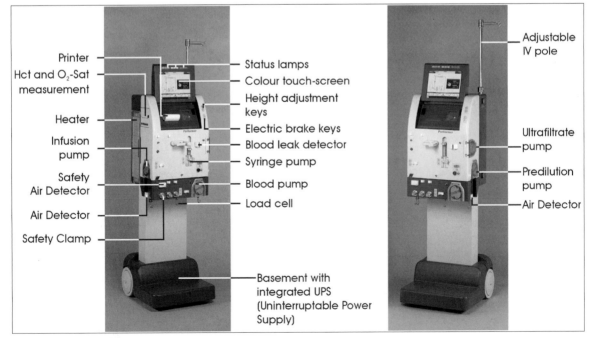

Figure 12.2: Main features.

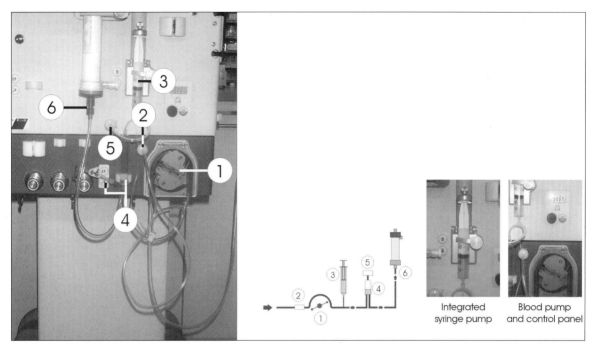

Figure 12.4: Blood circuit set-up: arterial line. 1. Mounting of pump segment (8 x12 mm section) into blood pump. 2. Connection to withdrawal pressure transducer. 3. Syringe pump (20, 30 ml syringe can be mounted). 4. Expansion chamber (with automatic level regulation) to collect air before the filter. 5. Connection to pre-filter pressure transducer. 6. Connection of arterial line to the filter's in-flow blood port.

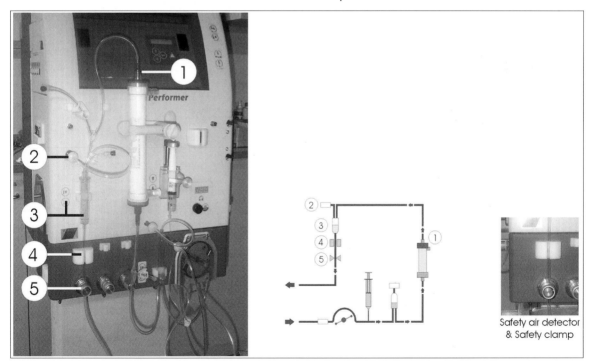

Figure 12.5: Blood circuit set-up: venous line. 1. Connection of venous line to the filter's out-flow blood port. 2. Connection to return pressure transducer. 3. Venous drip chamber (with automatic level regulation). 4. Safety air sensor (ultrasound type) to detect air bubbles in patient's return line. 5. Safety clamp to stop blood flow in case of air detection.

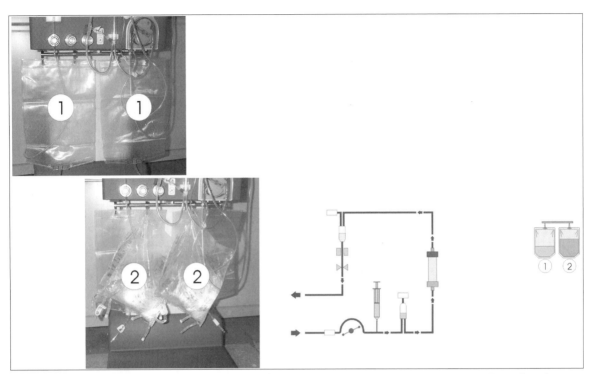

Figure 12.6: Fluid bags set-up. 1. Ultrafiltrate collecting bags hanging on scales. 2. Replacement solution bags hanging on scales (max load=20 liters).

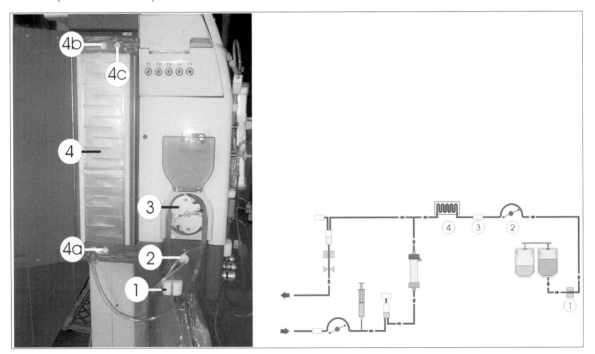

Figure 12.7: Replacement circuit set-up: infusion line. 1. Insertion of line into Air Sensor to detect fluid run out. 2. Connection to infusion pressure transducer. 3. Mounting pump segment into infusion pump. 4. Mounting heating bag into heater (plate type) to warm replacement fluid: 4a. Temperature sensor to measure inlet temperature of fluid. 4b.&4c. Temperature sensors to measure outlet temperature (control and protection sensor).

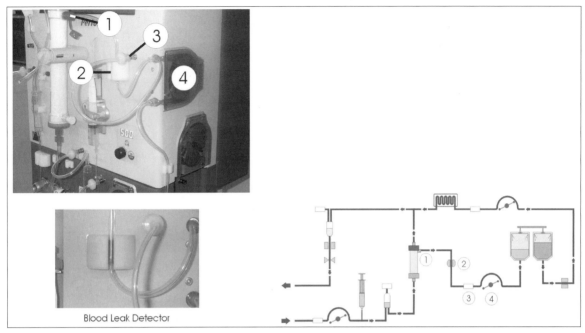

Figure 12.8: Replacement circuit set-up: ultrafiltrate line. 1. Connection of ultrafiltrate line to the filter's port.
2. Insertion of line into Blood Leak Detector to detect presence of blood in the ultrafiltrate (0.5% sensitivity).
3. Connection to ultrafiltrate pressure transducer. 4. Mounting of pump segment into ultrafiltrate pump.

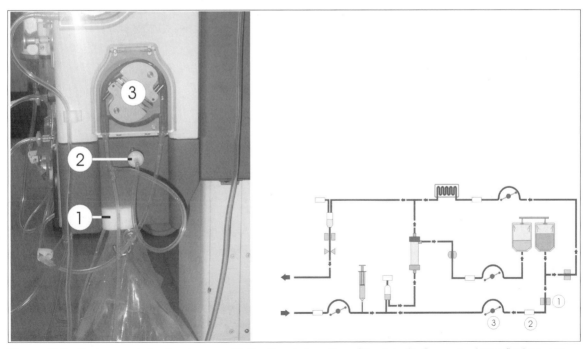

Figure 12.9: Replacement circuit set-up: predilution line. 1. Insertion of line into Air Sensor to detect fluid run out.
2. Connection to predilution pressure transducer. 3. Mounting of pump segment into predilution pump.

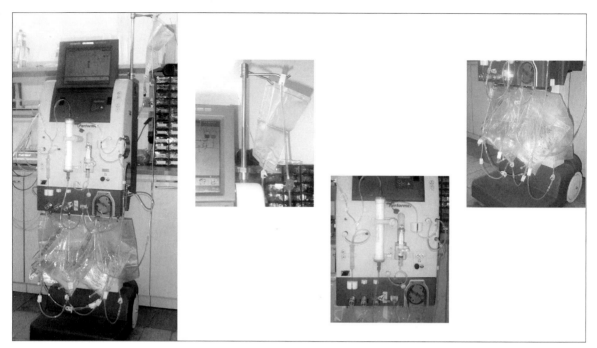

Figure 12.10: Equipment ready for priming and rinsing.

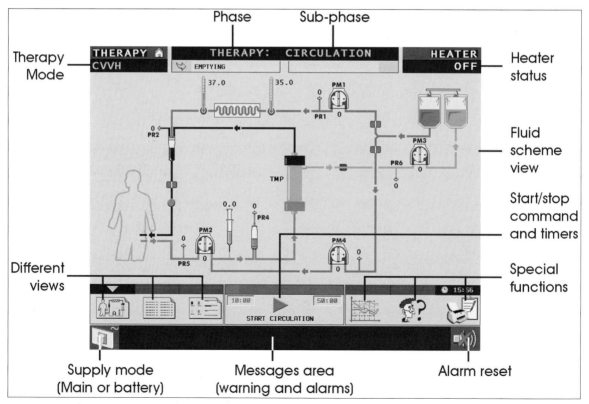

Figure 12.11: Example of a typical display view.

13

Pediatric CRRT

Barry Wilkins and Anne Morrison

Hemofiltration in children

Hemofiltration has been performed in infants and children since the early 1980s. Although there are some important differences in the indications, methods and parameters between children and adult patients, the technique is essentially the same. Arterio-venous circuits were first used, as in adults, and, although much simpler, have now been replaced by veno-venous circuits incorporating a blood pump. The latter technique produces much more reliable blood flow and filtrate flow and is theoretically better tolerated especially by patients with compromised circulation.

Indications include
1. Correction of water overload when the kidney is unable to excrete sufficient water.
2. To remove larger quantities of water from the body than the kidney is able to achieve in order to enable the administration of therapeutic fluids such as parenteral nutrition.
3. To remove excess electrolytes from the body in cases of retention of e.g. potassium, magnesium, phosphate.
4. Removal of urea and/or creatinine in cases of renal failure or hypercatabolic state where excess urea is produced.
5. Correction of disorders of acid/base homeostasis, particularly metabolic acidosis, when non-volatile acid is being produced in quantities greater than the kidney and liver can handle. A particularly important indication is for inborn errors of metabolism, which often present with severe intractable metabolic acidosis or aminoacidemia.
6. Occasionally, removal of ingested poisons or toxins in sepsis.

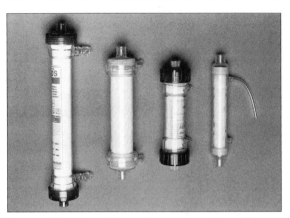

Figure 13.1: Hemofilters of various sizes from different manufacturers, suitable for CVVH or CVVHDF. Membranes are made of polyamide, polysulfone and acrylonitrile. Priming volume varies from 11 to 60 ml.

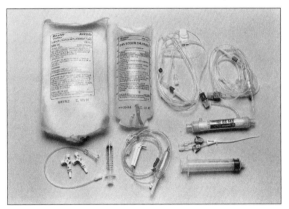

Figure 13.2: Equipment for setting up and priming the hemofiltration circuit. Note the narrow bore venous take-off and venous return lines, the small filter and the filtrate line and adaptor. A bag of saline with added heparin is to flush the circuit and filter.

Venous access in children is achieved using a double-lumen catheter. Either the femoral vein is used (but be careful that the catheter tip is in the lower end of the IVC, otherwise inadequate blood flow will result), or subclavian or internal or external jugular veins (tip at the SVC/R atrial junction).

As a general guide, use:

- 6.5 FG × 10 cm double lumen catheter in infants <10 kg
- 8 FG × 15 cm double lumen catheter in children 10–15 kg
- 11 FG × 20 cm double lumen catheter in children >15 kg

These will permit blood flows of at least 200, 300 and 400 ml/min respectively. The proximal lumen is usually for blood withdrawal (it is color coded red), the distal for blood return (blue). They can be interchanged if blood withdrawal is poor, but this may cause some recirculation of filtered blood through the circuit and consequently decreased clearances.

The narrower catheters are more prone to occlusion by thrombosis, so it is important to keep the lumens well flushed with heparin when there is no blood flow.

Children can be quite agitated in intensive care and are often resistant to sedation. Excessive patient movement may compromise blood flow if the femoral route is used. Avoid using any 3-way taps in the blood circuit as these greatly increase resistance within the circuit.

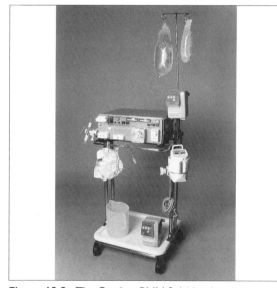

Figure 13.3: The Gambro BMM 3-1 blood pump machine. Note on the right the roller pump for blood flow. Two separate peristaltic pumps are for controlling the filtrate and the replacement fluid flow. The large jug is to collect the flushing (priming) fluid. A urine bag is used to collect the eventual filtrate when in operation. A heated coil warmer allows warming of the replacement fluid.

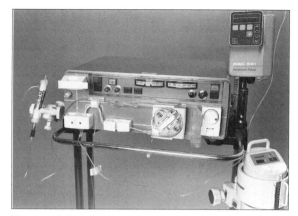

Figure 13.4: In this view the venous take-off line has been threaded through the roller blood pump and attached to one end of the hemofilter. The housing of the blood pump has been left temporarily open for clarity. Heparinized saline allows filling of the line and filter.

The blood pump illustrated is the Gambro AK10 system. Newer hemofiltration machines are coming on to the market but these are designed initially with adult patients in mind. Because they are microprocessor controlled, special software has to be designed to make them suitable for infants.

A problem with small children is the extracorporeal volume of blood. Generally it is wise to have less than 10% of the patient's blood in the circuit (i.e. <8 ml/kg) to avoid hemodynamic instability, although this latter can be avoided by paying careful attention to correcting hypovolemia beforehand, and the use of inotropes and vasopressors. Also, if a circuit clots rapidly before the circuit blood can be returned to the patient, then the patient will become rapidly anemic necessitating transfusions.

It is therefore important that the patient is fully anticoagulated before starting hemofiltration, and to maintain anticoagulation. There are a variety of methods. Heparinization with 20 units/kg/h, adjusted according to APTT or activated clotting time results, is the most popular method, but regional anticoagulation has been used, or citrate.

It has been the usual practice of prescribing a filtrate flow rate of 30–50 ml/kg/h in children. This is controlled by a separate pump, preferably a volumetric one, although the latter is often not available. Peristaltic pumps are inaccurate up to about 5% of the prescribed value. The filtrate volume is often less than prescribed. The filtrate can, however, be weighed each hour, and the volume of replacement fluid adjusted. This makes the process more labor intensive and meticulous attention to detail must be observed continuously. The replacement fluid volume is also often less than prescribed because the peristaltic pump is delivering a high flow rate of fluid into a relatively high pressure system, especially if the replacement fluid is delivered postfilter.

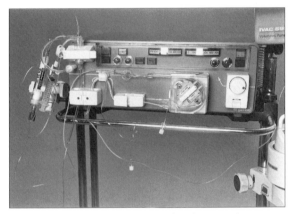

Figure 13.5: The venous return line has now been attached to the filter and bubble trap inserted into the air detector housing. A syringe and 3-way tap allows adjustment of the air/blood level in the bubble trap. Air detection is bypassed during the flushing procedure. The venous return line is loose in the sterile jug to collect the waste flushing fluid. The pressure sensing line from the top of the bubble trap has been attached to the pressure transducer nipple at the very left of the machine. This allows monitoring of the venous return pressure.

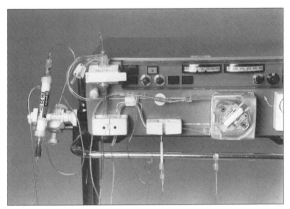

Figure 13.6: The filtrate line and replacement fluid line have now been attached and primed. In this view the replacement fluid has been attached to a side port in the venous takeoff line just before the blood pump, for pre-filter addition of the replacement fluid. It can be attached alternatively to the bubble trap for post-filter addition.

Filtrate flow of 30–50 ml/kg/h is greater than in adult patients. With any inaccuracies in delivery of filtrate and replacement fluid, a patient can develop water imbalance very rapidly. The commonest problem is for the patient to become progressively dehydrated, despite the fluid charts suggesting neutral balance. It is most important therefore that children on hemofiltration are examined frequently for clinical signs of fluid imbalance. Newer integrated volumetric pump systems should overcome these problems when they have been configured for use in infants and children.

Blood flow should be at least 6 times the filtrate flow, or at least 3 ml/kg/min for a filtrate of 30 ml/kg/h. The increased hematocrit which develops as blood flows through the filter can increase viscosity and hasten the failure of the filter membrane. Pre-filter addition of the replacement fluid avoids this problem, but clearance is reduced and there is no evidence of improved filter life.

The Gambro system illustrated allows the use of very narrow bore lines with an extracorporeal blood volume of only 27 ml when used with a small filter. The blood pump speed has to be corrected for the narrow bore of the pump segment of the circuit. Again, when pediatric circuits are developed for the new machines, this should no longer be a problem.

When hemofiltration is prescribed for inborn errors of metabolism, high clearance of organic acids or amino acids may be desirable. Hence, in this special case, higher filtration rates may be needed. It is possible to achieve up to 100 ml/kg/h, which more than equals the patient's normal glomerular filtration rate. Alternatively, or in addition, dialysis can be added (for example, 50 ml/kg/h filtrate plus 50 ml/kg/h dialysate, and 100 ml/kg/h of filter effluent). CVVHDF is generally not otherwise necessary in children and should be discouraged because it adds to the complexity.

The replacement fluid used in children has usually been a near physiological solution but with lactate as a bicarbonate substitute to improve shelf life. Mild degrees of hyperlactatemia occur and are of no consequence. However, in cases of lactic acidosis, and inborn errors of metabolism, and in hepatic failure, the lactate may not be metabolized. Regular monitoring of lactate or of anion gap is therefore necessary. This problem is solved by using a bicarbonate based replacement fluid which has to have the bicarbonate added immediately before use. This is more labor intensive but allows improved control of acid–base balance. With severe liver failure lactatemia may continue.

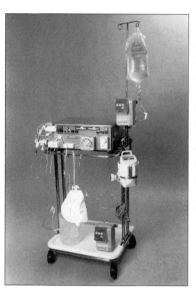

Figure 13.8: Overall view of fully prepared circuit. The only connection which is not yet complete is that of the ultrafiltrate line to the IV volumetric pump which will be used to control ultrafiltration rate.

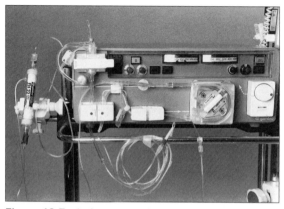

Figure 13.7: A closer view shows that the venous take-off and venous return lines have now been joined with a connector to allow circulation of priming fluid before connecting to the patient's double lumen central venous catheter. They have been coiled up in this view for clarity. The separate small coiled side connector is for the addition of heparin by a separate syringe pump.

14

Anticoagulation During CRRT

Rinaldo Bellomo and Claudio Ronco

Introduction

Anticoagulation is an important aspect of the care of patients receiving CRRT. The need for anticoagulation of the CRRT circuit arises from the fact that the contact between blood and the tubing of the circuit and the membrane of the filter induces activation of the coagulation cascade. This extracorporeal activation of the coagulation cascade inevitably results in filter or circuit clotting[1].

It is generally desirable to operate CRRT on a truly continuous basis (i.e. 24 hours/day). Such continuous operation ensures that adequate urea and creatinine clearances are achieved and maintained. It also ensures that a limited period of time is spent setting up and priming a new filter. Such setting up and priming activity is time-consuming. Typically, setting up the circuit can take from 0.5–1.5 hours depending on the circuit and the expertise of the nurses involved. In the intensive care unit such setting up is either performed by the ICU nurse or by the dialysis nurse. Both nurses are typically very busy delivering patient care. Having to take time off from such patient care is an important undesirable consequence of frequent circuit clotting. Thus, a major goal of anti-coagulation is to ensure smooth operation of the ICU and to minimize time spent changing the circuit (i.e. a 'practical' goal). If CRRT is run at minimal levels of clearance (15–17 ml/min of urea clearance), time spent off the filter will significantly decrease the clearance of uremic toxins and result in inadequate uremic control.

A second goal of anti-coagulation is to maintain adequate clearances. It is important to note, however, that in units (such as the author's) that run CRRT at a higher level of efficiency (urea clearance of 33 ml/min), some time spent 'off the filter', even hours, has little practical impact on uremic control. Such control remains very good (plasma [urea] <25 mmol/l at all times). To state this issue in another way, the impact of 'down time' on uremic control is clinically negligible if CRRT is run at higher clearances.

A third goal of anti-coagulation may be that of avoiding the generation of inflammatory substances from blood–membrane contact. The data supporting a degree of clinical significance for this third goal of anti-coagulation, however, are not available.

The fourth goal of anti-coagulation is to minimize the costs associated with CRRT. Each filter and circuit change can cost more than Aus$100 in disposables only. Using 3 instead of 6 circuits over a one week period results in considerable savings.

The fifth goal of anti-coagulation is to achieve all the above aims with minimal risk to the patient. In practice, however, any form of intervention aimed at prolonging circuit life is associated with some risk[2]. It important to note, however, that the overriding principle of anti-coagulation during CRRT should be that *losing the filter is better than losing the patient*. Under no circumstances should the patient's well being be put at unreasonable risk of bleeding just to prolong circuit life. This consideration is particularly important because, in the vast experience of the author, circuit failure is often due to vascular access inadequacy rather than insufficient circuit anti-coagulation. Thus, increasing anti-coagulation is often the incorrect therapeutic step (due to incorrect diagnosis of the cause of filter failure). Increasing anti-coagulation increases risk of bleeding and yet it may not resolve the problem of frequent circuit clotting.

Considerations related to techniques and patient features

Several technical features of the CRRT circuit are likely to influence the success of any approach to anti-coagulation. If an arterio-venous circuit is used, the most important variable in maintaining circuit patency is the quality of vascular access. The greater the blood flow rates the greater the statistical likelihood of prolonging circuit life. Thus, circuit life is longer with femoral cannulae compared to a Scribner shunt[3]. It is equally important that the tubing be as short as possible to decrease resistance to flow[4]. If a pumped system is used, some observations are of importance to filter life. First, the 'set' pump speed may be inaccurate (NB: typically the value displayed reflects the 'systolic' pump speed, not the 'mean' pump speed). Secondly, in cases of catheter kinking, patient positional changes, or nursing intervention, there may be significant flow fluctuations with reductions in real flow of >50%. Such reductions may occur without any alarms warning the operator that actual flow has seriously declined. The pump may continue to rotate, but actual blood flow may be little if any at all. Such unrecognized stasis of blood in the circuit can last for several minutes and will increase the chance of circuit clotting. The problem under these circumstances is related to inadequate vascular access (access failure). Such access failure may be acute (previously reasonably functioning access which has become kinked or is abutting the wall of the vein and cannot deliver blood to the circuit); chronic (partially clotted orifices or lumen with chronic difficulty in delivering the set flow); or acute on chronic.

If the incorrect diagnosis is made (i.e. circuit clotting due to failure of anti-coagulation is diagnosed instead of access failure-related clotting), the intensity of anti-coagulation is then stepped up. Such an approach to prolonging filter life under these circumstances is often futile. Furthermore, it is always dangerous to the patient who becomes unnecessarily exposed to an increased risk of bleeding.

Another common site of clotting is the venous 'bubble trap'. Air/blood contact promotes clotting. Furthermore, the additional contact with plastic and a degree of stasis (transit time for the cellular elements is often prolonged by eddies within the bubble trap) also promote intra-chamber clotting. In a recent in-house study at the author's institution, >20% of circuit failures were due to clot within the bubble trap.

It is possible that the type of membrane makes a difference to circuit life[5] as may be the case with filter geometry[6] but the data available is limited in quality and quantity. Furthermore, the general observation is that pumped systems last for a shorter period of time compared with spontaneous systems. Also, systems with high filtration fractions have shorter operational lives and systems operating with post-dilutional fluid replacement may also have a shorter duration of operation than CRRT with pre-dilutional fluid replacement[1,7,8].

Finally, if heparin is the anticoagulant of choice, it appears that administration of a more dilute heparin solution may improve filter life[9].

There are also patient features, which play an important role in determining circuit life. Some obvious clinical features include the presence of endogenous coagulopathies (liver disease, hemophilia) and thrombocytopenia. In the presence of such risk factors for bleeding, filter life can often be prolonged even in the absence of any circuit anti-coagulation. Less well appreciated is the effect that antithrombin III (ATIII) deficiency can have on filter life. Many septic patients, cardiac surgery patients or liver patients have marked ATIII deficiency. Such ATIII deficiency strongly predisposes to filter clotting[10,11] and decreases the efficacy of heparin (ATIII is the co-factor for heparin). The administration of ATIII (thousands of dollars) can improve filter life but the cost of ATIII is much higher than that of filters (hundreds of dollars). Occasionally, sufficient ATIII replacement can be achieved with the administration of fresh frozen plasma. Such administration may paradoxically prolong filter life. The risk benefit ratio of such an approach is unknown.

Anticoagulants

Several anticoagulants are available to prolong filter life. They will be reviewed here in some detail.

Heparin
This agent is the most commonly available anticoagulant[3]. It is easy to use and clinicians are extremely familiar with its use. It can be used in different ways as described below.

1) *Low-dose pre-filter heparin*: In the author's unit this dose is any dose less than 5 IU/kg/h. This dose typically does not have any detectable effect on activated partial thromboplastin time (aPTT), international normalized ratio (INR) or activated clotting time (ACT). We use this in most of our patients as it appears safe and likely to prolong filter life. There are, however, no controlled studies to confirm such an effect.

2) *Medium-dose pre-filter heparin*: This expression indicates a heparin dose of 8–10 IU/kg/h. Such a dose often results in a mild prolongation of aPTT (10–20% in most cases). We use this approach in patients with little risk of bleeding who may require a degree of prophylactic anticoagulation anyway, or who may have had limited filter lives with lower heparin doses (provided that vascular access dysfunction has been excluded).

3) *Systemic heparinization*: This dose is reserved for patients who require systemic anticoagulation for other reasons (pulmonary embolism, valve replacement). In the author's unit, this dose is never used just to prolong filter life.

4) *Regional heparinization*: This approach describes the use of pre-filter heparin at doses expected to induce systemic anticoagulation but associated with the post-filter administration of protamine to reverse its anticoagulant effect[12,13]. Typically, we start with 1500 IU/h of pre-filter heparin and administer 10–12 mg/h of post-filter protamine. Protamine is administered as close to the end of the circuit as possible to maximize the effects of heparin on the circuit and minimize its effects on the patient. This approach is usually monitored by studying the patient's aPTT. The aPTT should be slightly prolonged at most. This approach has been shown to prolong filter life when blood flow is slow[3]. We use it in patients who have very limited circuit duration despite seemingly adequate vascular access.

5) *Low molecular weight heparins (LMWH)*: These newer agents can be effectively used to prolong filter life even though they have not been shown to be superior to heparin in this regard[14]. The dose should be adjusted to the clinical situation and the type of LMWH used. Monitoring of anticoagulation with LMWH is more cumbersome and reversal with protamine only partial. These agents are also more expensive than standard heparin. They may be tried in some cases of heparin-induced thrombotic thrombocytopenia. However, cross reactivity occurs in >90% of cases and low molecular weight heparinoids are preferable.

6) *Low molecular weight heparinoids*: Rarely, patients who receive hemofiltration with heparin anticoagulation develop heparin-induced thrombotic thrombocytopenia syndrome (HITTS). When HITTS develops the circuit clots repeatedly and the patient is at simultaneous risk of bleeding and thrombosis. Under these circumstances, heparinoids have been shown to have minimal (<10%) cross-reactivity and to represent a reasonable alternative for the purpose of circuit anticoagulation[15].

Prostacyclin (PGI$_2$)

This agent is potentially useful for the purpose of circuit anticoagulation because of its effect on platelets. In fact, prostacyclin is the most potent inhibitor of platelet aggregation yet discovered and has been reported to be effective by several groups[16]. It is unknown whether it is more effective than heparin. Langenecker and co-workers[17] found no significant difference in filter life when they compared prostacyclin at close to 8 ng/kg/min with heparin at 6 IU/kg/h[17]. However, prostacyclin administration induced hypotension. When they combined prostacyclin (5 ng/kg/min) with heparin (6 IU/kg/h) they prolonged filter life from 14 to 22 hours. Thus prostacyclin may be useful in prolonging filter life or as an alternative to heparin. However, reversal of its anticoagulant effect requires administration of fresh platelets and is therefore a more cumbersome and costly effort in patients receiving prostacyclin. Furthermore, the cost of 24 hours of prostacyclin infusion, even at doses of only 5 ng/kg/min, is in the range of US$100 (i.e. more expensive than a filter change). We rarely use prostacyclin for circuit anticoagulation.

Citrate

Citrate anticoagulation is a form of regional anticoagulation that depends on the ability of citrate to chelate calcium. The chelation of calcium prevents clot formation[1]. The method described by Mehta's group for CVVHDF can be modified to apply to CVVH. In brief, the procedure requires that a special calcium-free and sodium citrate-containing replacement solution and/or dialysate solution be prepared and administered at the appropriate rate to achieve the desired ACT (200–250 seconds) or aPTT (60–90 seconds). Calcium chloride is then administered separately to replace chelated, dialyzed calcium and maintain normacalcemia. This approach to anticoagulation is effective in maintaining excellent filter patency rates and compares favorably with heparin. It also avoids the risk of heparin-induced thrombocytopenia and does not lead to systemic anticoagulation. Drawbacks of this approach include the risk of hypocalcemia, the incidence of metabolic alkalosis (approximately 25%), and the cumbersome nature of dialysate/replacement fluid preparation. In the USA, where commercially available sterile solutions for CVVH/D are not available yet, such fluid preparation may not be a greater problem than the preparation of other fluids.

Nafamostat mesilate or gabexate mesilate

These agents are serine proteinase inhibitors and have been used to achieve circuit anticoagulation in dialysis and hemofiltration, particularly in Japan[18]. Such agents are expensive and not yet widely available in the USA, Europe or Australia. They appear to be at least as effective as heparin and perhaps associated with a lesser risk of bleeding.

No anticoagulation

In patients at risk of bleeding, it is possible to provide CRRT without anticoagulation and yet achieve acceptable filter lives (20–24 hours). This approach to 'anticoagulation' is obviously the safest for the patient. Indeed, we do not use any anticoagulant in patients who have a platelet count of <50 000, an INR >2, an aPTT >60 seconds or who are actively bleeding or have

had a recent (last 24 hours) bleeding episode. In selected patients who do not quite have such abnormalities of anticoagulation, we may also apply no anticoagulation on the basis of clinical judgement and the result of an initial 'trial of no anticoagulation'. The reasonable results achieved with such an approach have been reported[3]. This approach is frequently used in patients with liver diseases, either in the setting of fulminant liver failure/chronic liver failure with variceal bleeding or following liver transplantation. Another group of patients where this approach is acceptable and safe is one that includes patients with severe ARF following cardiac surgery or receiving extracorporeal membrane oxygenation. It is important to note that such an approach is predicated on the availability of adequate vascular access and the maintenance of good blood flows (preferably >250 ml/min).

Other approaches to prolonging filter life

Beyond the traditional anticoagulant-based approaches to maintaining filter life, several other strategies have also been tried. For example, coating of the filter with heparinized albumin has been suggested as a means of preventing fibrinogen binding, increasing membrane biocompatibility and prolonging filter life. Work by Reeves et al.[19], however, has shown this strategy to be ineffective. Low molecular weight dextran also has anticoagulant properties and may be useful in prolonging filter life. However, a controlled trial by Palevsky et al.[20] failed to shown any increase in filter life when dextran was used. Finally, several units use frequent saline flushes to remove procoagulant material from the filter on a regular basis. No large controlled study has been conducted to determine whether this strategy is effective in prolonging circuit life.

Monitoring anticoagulation

The need to monitor anticoagulation over and above the routine needs of critically ill patients simply because of CRRT is not clearly established. Because of our conservative approach to circuit anticoagulation, we often perform measurements of platelet count, aPTT and INR once a day. However, if regional anticoagulation is applied or systemic anticoagulation is achieved, such monitoring may become more frequent and occur two or three times daily. In a situation where citrate anticoagulation is applied, monitoring of calcium levels and ACT may occur 6-hourly. Thus when a clinician assesses the utility and cost of a given approach to anticoagulation, the following variables have to be factored in: cost of filter change; risk and morbidity of filter change; cost of anticoagulant; risk and morbidity of bleeding; and cost of monitoring. In each patient a careful judgement must be made on how one can achieve the best balance of risks and benefits in this aspect of patient care.

Summary

Maintenance of an acceptable filter life (24 hours or greater) is an important therapeutic goal during CRRT, but must not be sought at a significantly increased risk of bleeding for the patient. Various drugs and approaches are available to achieve the optimal balance between the risks and benefits of circuit anticoagulation in a given patient as illustrated above. Awareness and full understanding of all available options is the first step toward the correct choice.

References

1. Mehta R. Anticoagulation for continuous renal replacement therapies. In Ronco C, Bellomo R, eds. *Critical Care Nephrology*. Dordrecht; Kluwer academic Publishers: 1998: pp 1199–1211.
2. Ward DM, Mehta RL. Extracorporeal management of acute renal failure patients at high risk of bleeding. *Kidney Int* 1993; 43: S237–S244.
3. Bellomo R, Teede H, Boyce N. Anticoagulation regimen in acute continuous hemodiafiltration: a comparative study. *Intensive Care Med* 1993; 19: 329–332.
4. Jenkins R. The extra-corporeal circuit: physical principles and monitoring. In Ronco C, Bellomo R, eds. *Critical Care Nephrology*. Dordrecht, Kluwer Academic Publishers; 1998: pp 1189–1197.
5. Van de Wetering, Westendorp RGJ, van der Hoeven JG, Stolk B, Feuth JDM, Chang PC. Heparin use in continuous renal replacement procedures: the struggle between filter

coagulation and patient hemorrhage. *J Am Soc Nephrol* 1996; 7: 145–150.
6. Yohay DA, Butterly DW, Schwab SJ, Quarles LD. Continuous arteriovenous hemodialysis; effect of dialyzer geometry. *Kidney Int* 1992; 42: 448–451.
7. Favre H, Martin PY, Stoermann C. Anticoagulation in continuous extracorporeal renal replacement therapy. *Semin Dial* 1996; 9: 112–118.
8. Kaplan AA. The predilution mode for continuous arteriovenous hemofiltration. In Paganini E, ed. *Acute Continuous Renal Replacement Therapy*. Boston: Martinus Nijhoff; 1986: pp 143–146.
9. Golper TA. Indications, technical considerations and strategies for renal replacement therapy in the intensive care unit. *J Intensive Care Med* 1992; 7: 310–317.
10. Singer M, McNally T, Screaton G, Machin S, Cohen SL. Heparin clearance during continuous venovenous hemofiltration. *Intensive Care Med* 1994; 20: 212–215.
11. Bastien O, French P, Paulus S, et al. Antithrombin III deficiency during continuous venous hemodialysis. In Sieberth HG, Stummvoll HK, Kierdorf H, eds. *Continuous Extracorporeal Treatment in Multiple Organ Dysfunction Syndrome*. Basel: Contrib Nephrol, Karger; 1995: 116: 154–158.
12. Kaplan AA, Petrillo R. Regional heparinization for continuous arteriovenous hemofiltration. *Trans Am Soc Artif Intern Organs* 1987; 23: 312–315.
13. Maher JF, Lapierre L, Schreiner GE, Geiger M, Westerfelt FB Jr. Regional heparinization for hemodialysis. *N Engl J Med* 1963; 268: 451–456.
14. Wynckel A, Bernieh B, Toupance O *et al.* Guidelines for using enoxaparin in slow continuous hemodialysis. *Intensive Behandlung* 1990; 15: 117–119.
15. Magnani HN. Heparin-induced thrombocytopenia: an overview of 230 patients treated with orgaran. *Thromb Haemostasis* 1993; 70: 554–561.
16. Scheeren T, Radermacher P. Prostacyclin: new aspects of an old substance in the treatment of critically ill patients. *Intensive Care Med* 1997; 23: 146–158.
17. Langenecker SA, Falfernig M, Werba A, Mueller C, Chiari A, Zimpfer M. Anticoagulation with prostacyclin and heparin during condinuous

venovenous hemofiltration. *Crit Care Med* 1994; 22: 1774–1781.

18. Hu ZJ, Iwama H, Suzuki R, Kobayashi S, Akutsu I. Time course of activated coagulation time at various sites during continuous haemodiafiltration using nafamostat mesilate. *Intensive Care Med* 1999; 25: 524–527.

19. Reeves JH, Seal P, Voss AL, O'Connor. Albumin priming does not prolong hemofilter life. *ASAIO J* 1997; 43: 193–196.

20. Palevsky PM, Burr R, Moreland L, Tokiwa Y, Greenberg A. Failure of low molecular weight dextran to prevent clotting during continuous renal replacement therapy. *ASAIO J* 1995; 41: 847–849.

15

Trouble-Shooting During CRRT: Clinical and Technical Problems

Rinaldo Bellomo, Ian Baldwin, Thomas Golper, Claudio Ronco

Introduction

The intensive care or nephrology physician or nurse who is prescribing or conducting CRRT is often faced with technical or clinical problems. Such is the nature of any therapy that is intended to run for 24 hours a day in an environment like the intensive care. In such an environment the patient's clinical condition and position change frequently as do the physician's therapeutic goals. The same is true of vascular access performance, circuit function and machine function. To help CRRT practitioners we have assembled a series of cases that illustrate some clinical and technical problems we have faced in our experience of more than 1000 cases, and some of the solutions we have found for such problems. The solutions provided are not the only approach to trouble-shooting in a particular situation. We hope, however, that these case histories will assist CRRT practitioners in developing a view of their own on how best to solve the practical problems that face them every day as they seek to offer their patients the safest and most effective form of renal support.

Case 1

A 20-year-old man was admitted to the ICU 3 days after trans-sphenoidal surgery for nasopharyngeal carcinoma. He had been stable until 12 hours earlier but had now developed a fever of 40°C, unresponsive to paracetamol, a deterioration in conscious state from a Glasgow Coma Score of 14 to 9 and severe hypernatremia ([Na] = 156 mmol/l). His serum creatinine was normal. His urine output was 200 ml/h. The CT scan showed blood in the ventricular system (no change from previous scan) and cerebral edema.

He was started on antibiotics, admitted to intensive care and intubated.

Problem: How can we correct this man's hypernatremia and hyperthermia without worsening his cerebral edema?

Response: By using hemofiltration, which will slowly and reliably lower serum sodium and body temperature.

A Camino intra-cranial pressure monitoring device was inserted. A femoral double-lumen catheter was inserted. Hemofiltration (CVVH) was initiated at 2 l/h exchanges. CVVH was conducted without anticoagulation because of the perceived risk of bleeding. IV steroids were administered. Twenty-four hours later, the serum sodium has fallen to 143 mmol/l, the body temperature from 40°C to 37.2°C, and the intracranial pressure from 24 mmHg to 12 mmHg. All values remained essentially stable for another 24 hours with continued CVVH. The filter lasted 42 hours. The patient woke up and was extubated and discharged from ICU 2 days later and from the hospital 8 days later. He had a full recovery.

Case 2

A 65-year-old woman had been in the ICU for 8 days with ARDS following aspiration pneumonia on day one after gastrectomy. Her chest X-ray showed persistent bilateral infiltrates, her PaO_2 was 73 mmHg on an FiO_2 of 0.85. Her positive end expiratory pressure (PEEP) was 12 cm H_2O. A pulmonary artery catheter showed a right atrial pressure (RAP) of 16 mmHg, a pulmonary artery occlusion pressure (PAOP) of 17 mmHg and a cardiac index of 3.6 l/m²/min. Her mean atrial pressure (MAP) was 75 mmHg on a continuous norepinephrine infusion at 0.1 µg/kg/min. Sacral pitting edema was noted. An assessment was made that fluid overload was contributing to her ARDS. A furosemide infusion was started. Urine output was maintained at 150 ml/h. However, 24 hours later, she required 10 g of potassium replacement. Her serum potassium was 3.1 mmol/l and her serum sodium had risen from 142 mmol/l to 154 mmol/l. Her serum urea had changed from 15 mmol/l to 19 mmol/l. No changes in RAP or PAOP were noted.

Problem: How do we correct the suspected fluid overload, while avoiding hypokalemia and hypernatremia?

Response: By using hemofiltration, which will remove isotonic fluid and can be used to correct serum potassium.

A femoral catheter was inserted and CVVH was started. 20 mmol of potassium were added to her 5-liter commercial replacement fluid bags, which only contain 1 mmol/l of potassium. Anticoagulation was with heparin at 800 IU/h. CVVH fluid balance was kept at −300 ml/h. Twenty-four hours later, her fluid balance was negative by 3.8 l. Her RAP was 10 mmHG and her PAOP was 12 mmHg. Her serum [Na] was 138 mmol/l and the serum [K] was 4.4 mmol/l. Her PaO_2 was 89 mmHg and the FiO_2 was 0.5. CVVH was continued for another 24 hours and another 2.3 l of isotonic fluid was removed with a further improvement in oxygenation. She was extubated 2 days later.

Case 3

A 53-year-old man had undergone a pericardectomy for constrictive pericarditis. He had a malfunctioning renal transplant with chronic rejection and renal failure. His urine output was maintained and his pre-surgery urea was 26 mmol/l. Prior to surgery he was given desmopressin acetate (DDAVP) intravenously and 5 units of cryoprecipitate. Surgery was undertaken with aprotinin cover. Nonetheless, significant bleeding from the pericardial granulation tissue complicated the operation despite the administration of clotting factors and platelets. When the patient was admitted to the cardiothoracic ICU his chest drainage was 300 ml/h. His INR was 2.3, his aPTT was 65 seconds, his Hb was 84 g/l, and his platelet count was 56 000/mm³. His cardiac

index was 2.4 l/m²/m. His PAOP was 20 mmHg and his chest film showed early pulmonary edema. His urine output had declined to 20 ml/h despite the administration of 250 mg of furosemide. The cardiac surgeon indicated that he would not take the patient back to theater because the bleeding was 'medical' and could not be stopped by any surgical intervention.

Problem: How do we correct this patient's coagulopathy, anemia, and thrombocytopenia without inducing massive pulmonary edema?

Response: By simultaneously performing hemofiltration and maintaining a near neutral fluid balance

A femoral catheter was inserted and the patient was started on CVVH. In the ensuing 8 hours he received the following blood products: 10 units of fresh frozen plasma, 20 units of platelets, 20 units of cryoprecipitate, 5 units of packed red cells (total volume = 5.8 l). CVVH was performed without anticoagulation with a blood flow rate of 250 ml/min and a negative fluid balance of 500 ml/h. Chest drain losses decreased to 30 ml/h. The INR was 1.2, the aPTT was 39 seconds, the platelet count was 107 000/mm³ and the Hb was 102 g/l. The cumulative fluid balance for the 8 hour period was +8 ml. Hemofiltration was continued for another 2 hours at an even fluid balance. The circuit clotted after 10 hours of function. Hemofiltration was discontinued. The patient was extubated the following morning and discharged from the cardiothoracic ICU 36 hours after surgery.

Case 4

A 40-year-old woman was admitted to the ICU with fulminant liver failure from taking Chinese herbs. She was comatose and had to be immediately intubated. Her circulation was unstable and there was concern about aspiration pneumonia. A pulmonary artery catheter showed a cardiac index of 5.4 l/m²/min. A norepinephrine infusion was started to maintain a MAP of 70 mmHg. The infusion had to be rapidly escalated to maintain her blood pressure. After 8 hours in the ICU, her right pupil was seen to enlarge. Mannitol was immediately administered and a Camino intracranial pressure monitoring device was inserted. Her ICP was 34 mmHg.

Controlled hyperventilation was instituted and a CT scan was performed. The scan showed cerebral edema and a small subdural hematoma at the site of the intracranial pressure monitor insertion. Her ICP remained elevated at 25 mmHg despite further mannitol and then hypertonic saline treatment and a $PaCO_2$ of 33 mmHg. To maintain a cerebral perfusion pressure of >60 mmHg, her norepinephrine infusion had to be increased to 1.2 µg/kg/min. Her INR was 2.2 and her platelet count was 45 000/mm³. She had been anuric from admission to the ICU. Her temperature was 39°C.

Problem: How to provide tailored renal replacement therapy to this patient.

Response: A number of practical adjustments have to be made to safely initiate and conduct hemofiltration in this patient.

A femoral double lumen catheter was inserted under platelet (5 units) and FFP (5 units) cover. To avoid swings in intravascular filling or any hypotension upon initiating CVVH, the blood pump was initially switched on at a flow rate of only 25 ml/min. More FFP was administered at a similar rate to maintain filling and the norepinephrine infusion rate was increased to achieve a MAP of 90 mmHg before the start of CVVH. The blood path tubing slowly filled up with blood without the cerebral perfusion pressure falling below 60 mmHg. Approximately 7–8 minutes later, the blood had filled the tubing and filter and had returned to the patient. The peristaltic pump speed was then increased to 50 ml/min, then to 100, 150 and 200 ml/min over a period of 2–3 min. No anticoagulant was used at any time. Once the blood flow had been established and the patient had remained stable, hemofiltration was started. Any excessive volume that may have been given could now be gently removed. This extraordinarily unstable patient had been placed on CVVH with no hint of hypotension. CVVH was subsequently conducted at a blood flow rate of 250 ml/min and without anticoagulation. The first filter had to be replaced 46 hours later.

Case 5

A 69-year-old patient was admitted to the ICU with acute renal failure and septic shock due to intra-abdominal sepsis following colorectal surgery. He was obese and had a distended abdomen with an intra-abdominal pressure of 23 cmH_2O. He was started on CVVH at 1 l/h via a 13.5 Fr dual lumen femoral catheter with heparin anticoagulation at 500 IU/h and a blood flow of 150 ml/min via a Prisma machine. His first filter lasted only 12 hours. A second filter was placed *in situ* but it only lasted 8 hours. Anticoagulation was increased to 1200 IU of heparin/h and yet his third filter lasted only 6 hours. A fourth circuit was started.

Problem: How can we increase filter life to acceptable levels in this patient

Response: We need to understand the etiology of filter clotting. Only after we have made the correct diagnosis, we can take the appropriate steps.

In our experience, filter failure is often due to inadequacies of vascular access. Testing the adequacy of vascular access can be achieved by aspirating blood from the 'arterial' limb or injecting saline through the 'venous' limb. This testing, however, is not possible if the circuit is running. The Prisma machine, however, displays the pressures necessary to 'suck' blood from the 'arterial' limb and to return it via the 'venous' limb. At a blood flow of 180 ml/min (maximum blood flow rate with this device) the negative pressure applied to the 'arterial' lumen is usually in the range of 60–80 mmHg for the catheter in question. In this patient, 120 mmHg of negative pressure had to be applied and intermittent 'failure to deliver blood flow' occurred with the machine alarming and stopping. The diagnosis of moderately severe access disfunction was made. It was hypothesized that abdominal distention was contributing to it by compressing the pelvic-abdominal venous system. The catheter was moved to the internal jugular vein. The next filter was anticoagulated at only 500 IU of heparin/h and lasted 28 hours. The femoral catheter was guide wire exchanged into a four-lumen central line for extra IV access and to prevent any significant bleeding from its site.

Case 6

A 62-year-old woman had been treated with CVVH for 3 days for acute renal failure and septic shock secondary to penumonia. Filter life had been acceptable (>20 hours per filter) using a blood flow of 200 ml/min from an AK 10 Gambro blood module, a filtration rate of 2 l/h, a heparin infusion rate of 500 IU/h, and a 12 Fr double lumen catheter in the femoral position. During the night, however, 2 filters had clotted after only 3 hours. At 8 am, the ICU nurses had just connected another circuit and were ready to start therapy again while suggesting an increase in anticoagulation.

Problem: New onset of frequent filter clotting.
Response: Increasing anticoagulation may be the correct response, but first the correct diagnosis must be made and mechanical problems must be excluded.

The filter and circuit were connected and blood flow was started. The pump alarms were silent and the peristaltic pump was rotating. All seemed to be in order. However careful observation of a couple of air bubbles visible in the replacement fluid tubing was revealing. Such fluid and bubbles were supposed to enter the blood path in the pre-filter position, just 3 cm before the rotating cam of the pump. The careful observer could note, however, that such bubbles were not moving at all. They could not be pushed into the blood stream or sucked into it because of increased resistance. What was happening was that the peristaltic pump was rotating at the 'right' speed but blood was not being pumped out of the catheter, it was simply moving back and forth. Blood flow through the circuit was nil. However, because rotation was taking place and pressures were generated, no alarms were signalling that something was wrong. The circuit was disconnected and the arterial limb of the catheter was tested with a syringe. No blood could be drawn. The arterial limb of the catheter was completely blocked. The correct diagnosis was vascular access failure, not inadequate circuit anticoagulation. A guide wire exchange was attempted but clot impeded the passage of the wire. The catheter was removed and showed complete occlusion of the outflow 'arterial' lumen with clot. A new catheter was inserted in the jugular position. The next circuit lasted 32 hours without any increase in anticoagulation.

Case 7

A patient with multiorgan failure from a motor vehicle accident was initiated on CVVH electively and early. The dual lumen catheter placement went well, there was no active bleeding, but there were numerous potential bleeding sites. Coagulation and platelet parameters were normal. CVVH was initiated using a Hospal BSM-22 machine and a F-60 dialyzer as the hemofilter. Heparin was administered as a 0.9% NaCl solution of 5 units/ml at a rate of 50 ml/h, as a form of predilution. The absolute rate was 250 units/h. No initial bolus was administered. Blood flow was 250 ml/min and UFR was 2 l/h. Hematocrit was 35%. All substitution fluid was administered predilutionally. After 3 hours of operation the venous pressure rose from 50 to 80 mgHg. Nothing else appeared to change.

What should one do at this point?

There are several options. One is to do nothing, which in fact is what was done. That's why we have this case to discuss. What should have been done was to examine the venous drip chamber for potential clotting, the most likely cause of a rise in venous pressure. Any occlusion in the return system will raise the venous pressure, so most clinicians would evaluate the most common problem first, clotting in the venous chamber at the air–blood interface. Had this been done, a small clot would have been detected. At that point, the lines should have been aggressively flushed, at the very least or perhaps even changed. If there was no bleeding and the systemic aPTT was normal, then there is an option to increase the heparin a little. The plan to keep the systemic aPTT normal is sound because of the fear of bleeding from the numerous injuries. There are several ways to increase the heparin. One would be to increase the rate of the current drip from 50 to 100 ml/h. This will increase the absolute amount from 250 to 500 units/h. During CVVH with a UFR of 2 l/h, we try to keep the heparin drip always at a rato of at least 100 ml/h to mix well with the inflowing blood. So this drip was too slow to begin with. If one did not want to increase the absolute amount of heparin, then dilute it further, to 2.5 units/ml, but have heparin dripping into the inflowing extracorporeal blood at all times. A UFR as high as 2 l/h easily accommodates a heparin infusion rate of

100 ml/h. We try to keep the heparin infusion to between 100–200 ml/h and simply change the concentration from 2.5 to 25 units/ml (solutions of 1 l of 0.9% NaCl plus 2500 to 25 000 units of heparin). The most frequently used solutions are 5000 or 10 000 units in 1 l of saline.

The use of predilution substitution fluid and a relatively low filtration fraction are filtration operating conditions compatible with attempting to use little anticoagulation. The predilution dilutes hematocrit, reducing sludging within the distal fibers, and dilutes the concentration of clotting proteins. The low filtration fraction does the same thing. In veno-venous systems it is prudent to keep the filtration fraction below 40% and in A-V systems below 20%. If that cannot be achieved with adequate solute removal, then hemofiltration should be diminished and dialysis added. Dialysis removes solute by diffusion and does not require dehydration of the blood, which promotes clotting.

What happened to this patient was that the filter completely clotted a few hours later and the entire scenario was repeated, with nothing corrected until the second filter clotted. At this point, CVVH had been running about 12 hours and the third filter was being used. The heparin drip was doubled in rate, and the filters lasted 24 to 30 hours for the next few days. No bleeding occurred and the aPTT never rose over 50 seconds. After 5 days of CVVH without further complications, hemodynamics gradually improved enough to tolerate regular hemodialysis at a rate of 5 sessions per week

Case 8

An anuric CVVH patient who was highly catabolic, weighed 60 kg, and had a total body water volume of 36 l, required a water exchange of 36 l/day to keep the BUN in an acceptable range (i.e. requires a daily Kt/V of 1.0). To achieve this the target UFR was set at 2 l/h or 33 ml/min, because there was inevitably some down time in the performance of the CVVH. Gentamicin was being given for an abdominal infection. A loading dose of 120 mg was given.

How should the antibiotic be dosed and monitored?

Because of its clearance predominantly by glomerular filtration, renal failure markedly decreases the clearance of gentamicin. Renal failure does not alter other pharmacokinetic parameters of this drug. Edema alters its volume of distribution because the aminoglycoside class actually does truly distribute into the extracellular water (sodium) space. Edema is not unique to renal failure. Therefore, the loading dose of gentamicin will be the same as in any edematous person. Most clinicians would administer a loading dose of 2 mg/kg to achieve a peak plasma concentration of 8 mg/l. If there is substantial edema, this dose will not quite achieve the desired peak. Give that dose and measure a peak level to corroborate that you are in the range of 6–10 mg/l desired for a peak. It is the peak level for aminoglycosides that reflect its antimicrobial effect. CVVH as renal replacement only enters the picture after the loading dose. CVVH will reproduce some fraction of artificial renal clearance. With a UFR of 33 ml/min this can act like a GFR of the same amount. One could use tables to see what recommendations are made for this GFR. About 40% of a usual maintenance dose is recommended every 12 hours.

Another approach is to estimate the amount removed and specifically replace that amount. This could be done by measuring the concentration of gentamicin in the filtrate at the halfway point of the dosing interval (as the average) and then multiply that average concentration by the filtrate volume to determine the amount lost into the filtrate during that dosing interval. Replace that amount. A variation of this approach utilizes blood levels to estimate the loss into filtrate. The mean of the peak and trough levels will reflect the average blood level during the dosing interval, since the elimination follows first order kinetics. This mean blood level represents what the filter sees as an average over the dosing interval. The sieving coefficient for gentamicin is 0.8, which means that the concentration in the filtrate is 80% of that in the blood. Thus, 80% of the mean blood level will approximate the concentration of gentamicin in the filtrate for that dosing interval. The volume of filtrate during the dosing interval × the mean filtrate concentration will approximate the absolute amount of gentamicin removed by CVVH. Replace that amount.

However, if we are going to obtain blood levels, let's use them directly to determine need, rather than to determine what was removed. The blood level is declining over time as the drug is removed by CVVH. The decline follows first order kinetics, so is linear if the clearance is stable, as it is during CVVH. Therefore, the average level over the dosing interval is the mean of the peak and trough levels, just as above. The peak level is 8 mg/l and a trough level 12 hours later is 2 mg/l. We can see clearly that the CVVH produced enough clearance such that the half life is 6 hours (one half life to go from 8 to 4 and a second half life to go from 4 to 2). To bring the level back up to the desired level of 8, the difference level (desired peak level – trough present level = difference level, in this example 8–2 = 6) is multiplied by the volume of distribution (0.25 l/kg) such that a supplemental dose of 90 mg is needed (6 mg/l × 0.25 l/kg × 60 kg = 90 mg). This approach establishes approximate half lives and replenishes the dose base on desired blood levels. This is the method I prefer when levels are available. When levels are not available, I prefer the estimations based on GFR.

Trouble-shooting CRRT: Nursing examples

The following examples are derived from an Australian data base of adverse events in the general ICU managing patients treated by CRRT. In each case the narrative entry from the incident is followed by a short discussion highlighting measures to minimize or prevent errors and complications.

Case 1
'A patient on CVVHD: Routine calculations of hourly fluid balance noticed that previous hours replacement not given; 720 ml. Patient was hemodynamically unstable – norepinephrine requirements increased. This occurred during shift change over'.

This problem implies that the fluid replacement was 'retrospective', with spontaneous ultrafiltrate formation and no pump control. This issue is eliminated with new machines where the ultrafiltrate loss is replaced concurrently or in a prospective manner. Replacing fluids lost in the previous hour in the current or next hour has the potential to render the patient hypovolemic.

Case 2
'Found Vas cath access lumen with air in it. Then noticed that air was pulsing in line above bubble trap. Vas cath lines clamped immediately and disconnected from CVVHD circuit. CXR and ABG performed on patient, no obvious problems. Vas cath line reinserted and CVVHD recommenced'.

Introduction of air into any extracorporeal circuit could have disastrous effects if the amount was significant. Air detector sensors are usually found on the return limb of machines for this reason. Most air tends to enter the circuit at any connections on the patient side of the roller pump (the tubing between the access catheter and the roller pump) where suction and negative pressure is greatest. Any connections here must be tight but not too tight to crack plastic connectors allowing air bubbles to be drawn in. A check of the connections, including the connection to the access should be part of any pre-patient connection check routine.

Case 3
'During set up of CVVH, power board with various pumps/heaters etc plugged into it was sitting on the tray under the CVVH machine. The 4 litre drainage bag was hanging in the usual position on the trolley. Power circuit breaker triggered and cut power to power board and machine. Power board found to have water in it. The drain bag was found to have a puncture in it and was leaking onto the tray'.

This incident highlights that using the BMM10-1 pump with IV pumps and a fluids warmer, mandates multiple power cord connections, usually into the one 'power board'. This helps with keeping the system electrically 'tidy' but means the power system must be kept clear of any fluid spills that may occur during priming or during use. Later custom built machines with integrated pumps and improved machine layout eliminate this. However even late model machines require waste fluids to collect into larger bags which can be a water–electrical hazard.

Case 4

'Patient required hemofiltration for acute renal failure, blood pressure supported by inotropes, to maintain SABP >90. Vas cath inserted, patient connected to hemofilter, within 30 seconds, blood pressure decreased to systolic 30; patient treated with epinephrine and responded. Blood pump ceased, patient further resuscitated with IV fluids from CVC line. CVVH circuit blood clotted'.

This event highlights that initiation of CVVH has the potential to cause sudden deterioration in the patient. Hypotension such as this will usually occur if the return limb of the circuit is not connected at start of treatment in the belief that the circuit volume will 'overload' the patient. This is often a practise in dialysis units, but is dangerous in the critically ill. Furthermore, any extra fluid can easily be removed by CRRT once the patient is stable. Both limbs of the access should be connected to the circuit and as blood is drawn from the patient, the dead space volume of the circuit is administered in return. In unstable, vasopressor-dependent patients, the saline being given as the blood enters the circuit will not sufficiently maintain intravascular volume. Intravascular volume depletion (acute venesection effect) will occur and hypotension will develop. Measures must be taken to prevent such events. Such measures include increasing the MAP prior to connection using a vasopressor dose increase, rapid fluid loading with 300–400 ml of colloid before initiating CRRT, or a minute or so before and during the first 3–5 minutes of CRRT, laying the patient flat at this time, and starting blood flow at a low rate (25 ml/min). It must be emphasized that it is foolish to initiate pump flow at 200 ml/min and acutely 'hemorrhage' 150–200 ml of blood out of a vasopressor-dependent patient. We have initiated CRRT in patients receiving >1 µg/kg/min of norepinephrine without even

the tiniest change in MAP. All one has to do is apply common sense and caution. All CRRT circuits should also have a saline flush line connected on the outflow limb ready for these events and to flush blood back to the patient when treatment is ceased.

Case 5

'CVVH functioning but venous return pressure very high (>250 mmHg) when blood pump speed increased above 100 ml/min immediately after connection of new circuit. Senior nurse asked to check system and noticed 3 way tap being used at connection of venous return line to vas cath. Previous 3 filters failed after 4, 7, and 1.5 hours associated with high venous pressure! Circuit using heparin (prefilter port) and protamine (post-filter into 3 way tap) – regional anticoagulation'.

This case example demonstrates the resistance to blood flow created by a 3-way tap being used in the blood path line. This resistance to blood flow means the blood flow cannot be increased without excessive pressure readings and filter clotting may result due to stasis of blood. If any drug or fluid needs to be administered into the return limb of the circuit it can be into the venous air chamber directly. Otherwise, a 'Y-piece' dialysis connector can be placed between the circuit and the access catheter. These connectors do not offer the resistance of a 3-way tap and normal blood flows are possible. The opening within a 3-way tap is little more than a 'pin' hole and is unsuitable for the rapid passage of blood. This case also highlights the need to make the correct 'diagnosis' when responding to frequent filter clotting.

Case 6

'A critically ill patient was commenced on CVVHDF at 2100 hours. At 2400 hours the patient blood temp had fallen from 36.2C to 34.8C. It was noted that there was no fluids warmer in line for the dialysate solution'.

Hemofiltration will cause hypothermia in most patients. This is worse in the CVVHDF mode where there is high exposure of patient blood to cool fluids due to the counter-current movement of the fluids and blood in the filter. In CVVH mode, fluids replacement in larger volumes (2 l/h) can also cause hypothermia. This adverse event indicates the need for a comprehensive treatment checklist routine prior to patient connection. New machines have a tubing circuit that makes it impossible not to have the fluids warmed prior to infusion. However, the option to have the warmer 'off' means that hypothermia can occur if the nurse fails to check for correct function. Note: there is no 'in line' temperature sensor-feedback system in any of the new machines.

16

Vascular Access for Continuous Renal Replacement Therapy

Rinaldo Bellomo and Claudio Ronco

Introduction

Adequacy of vascular access is perhaps the most important aspect of any extracorporeal therapy. It is particularly important in continuous renal replacement therapy where its performance is tested 24 hours a day. Under such circumstances, any inadequacies of access are sorely tested and frequently demonstrated. Such inadequacies are an important cause of circuit failure. A clear understanding of several practical aspects of vascular access is necessary for optimal and safe operation of any CRRT circuit.

Arterio-venous hemofiltration

This kind of CRRT requires cannulation of artery and vein. Such cannulation can be achieved by the creation of an arterio-venous shunt or by cannulation of the femoral vessels. The most common shunt for this purpose is an external silastic shunt described by Scribner. Such shunts have been almost completely abandoned because of the poor blood flow achieved and the risk of bleeding and complications. Femoral cannulation with suitably sized cannulae (size 13 or 14 Fr) can yield blood flows of 100 ml at a mean arterial pressure of 75–80 mmHg. Such flows are sufficient to achieve adequate volume removal by hemofiltration and adequate dialytic clearances if countercurrent low-flow dialysate is administered. Arterial cannulation in critically ill patients or in elderly patients with vascular disease is associated with a high degree of morbidity[1]. It is only justifiable in the field where pumps may not be available or in developing countries where pumps may be too expensive and thus only available in limited numbers or not available at all. We recommend that only veno-venous therapies be used.

Veno-venous hemofiltration

Veno-venous techniques rely on the use of a temporary double-lumen catheter. Such catheters are typically inserted into one of the central veins (Figure 16.1) (femoral, subclavian or jugular) by Seldinger technique[2]. Various designs (Figures 16.2 and 16.3) and brands are available, some incorporating a third lumen for drug infusion, others a peel-off insertion technique, others the combination of two separate catheters, and others again requiring a stylet for insertion. Their internal designs also differ (Figure 16.4, 16.5 and 16.6). Cuffed catheters for subcutaneous tunnelling are also available. However, their use in ICU patients is undesirable as the suspicion of sepsis frequently arises in critically ill patients. Under such circumstances, the physician is disadvantaged if he or she is using a catheter that cannot be easily removed or guide wire exchanged[3].

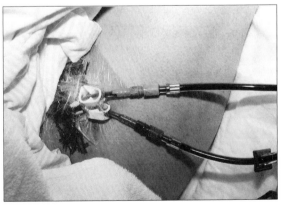

Figure 16.1: Photograph of a double lumen catheter inserted into the femoral vein.

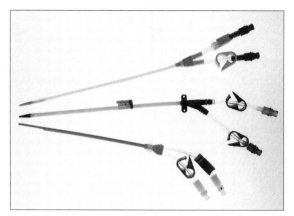

Figure 16.2: Photograph of three different double-lumen catheters used for CRRT.

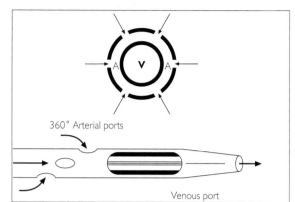

Figure 16.5: Diagram illustrating blood flow through a circumferential design catheter.

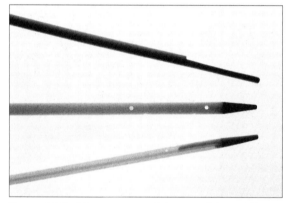

Figure 16.3: Close-up view of the tips of three different double-lumen catheters.

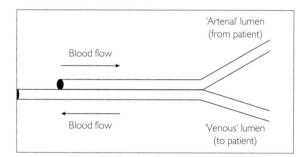

Figure 16.6: Diagram illustrating blood flow through two separate parallel channels. Such channels can be part of a single catheter or represent two separate single lumen devices inserted in parallel.

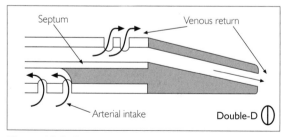

Figure 16.4: Diagram illustrating blood flow through a catheter with a double D luminal design.

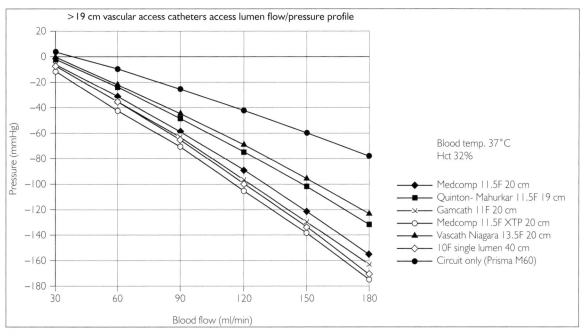

Figure 16.7: Diagram illustrating the amount of negative pressure that has to be applied to a variety of catheters to obtain a given blood flow through the 'aterial' lumen to obtain blood from the patient. As can be seen, not all catheters pose the same resistance to flow. The Niagara (Bard, Canada) catheter offers the least resistance to outflow.

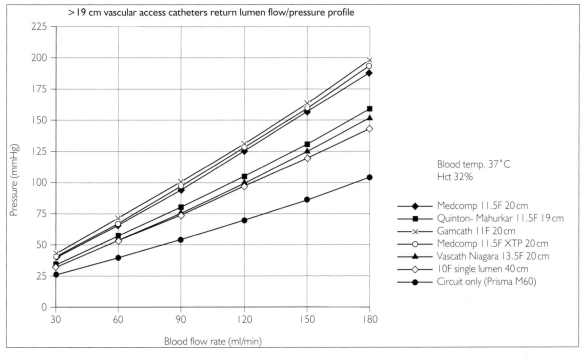

Figure 16.8: Diagram illustrating the amount of pressure that has to be applied to return a given amount of blood flow to the patient via the 'venous' limb of the catheter. As can be seen, different catheters offer different resistance to venous return.

Which catheter?

There is no controlled data comparing different types of catheters and their performance during CRRT. Such catheters can, however, be tested *in vitro* by creating an artificial CRRT circuit. A measure of their effectiveness is the resistance to flow for the arterial lumen and for the venous lumen. The 'resistance to outflow' can be tested by measuring the negative pressure that must be applied to achieve a certain flow through the 'arterial' limb of the catheter. Measuring how much positive pressure must be applied to achieve a certain flow through the 'venous' limb of the catheter can test the 'resistance to inflow'. We have conducted such tests *in vitro* (Figures 16.7 and 16.8) and have clearly demonstrated that catheters are different in their performance depending on their design, length and size.

Such *in vitro* testing, however, does not tell the full story. It is not useful to have a catheter that can reasonably easily yield 200 ml/min of blood flow rate *in vitro* but fails to do so *in vivo*. One reason for such discrepancies may lie in the design of the catheter. Side holes for 'arterial' outflow tend to suck the vessel walls against the

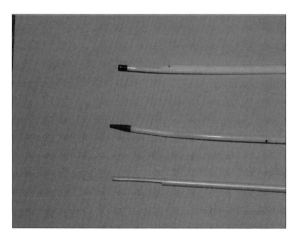

Figure 16.9: Photograph of three different catheters commonly used in our unit. The Niagara (blunt black tip) catheter has the biggest diameter (13.5 Fr) but its tip is hard. The Mahurkar has a sharp tip but a smaller diameter (11.5 Fr), which makes it suitable for smaller adult patients (weight <50 kg). The Cook catheter has a soft tip which permits its placement in the right atrium, if necessary. The Niagara catheter offers the least resistance to flow because of its size.

catheter thus paradoxically obstructing flow as more flow is asked for and greater negative pressure applied. Catheters that are too short and are inserted in the femoral position often only reach the external iliac vein. The flow of such a vein may only be 100–120 ml in the average human at rest. Asking for greater flows will require a suck back effect from the contralateral vein, which may not be possible with side-holed catheters. Longer catheters may offer more resistance to flow *in vitro* but, if inserted femorally, will reach the inferior vena cava and perform well *in vivo*. Our preference goes to large catheters (13.5 Fr) without side holes (Figure 16.9) and of a length (>20 cm) that allows the tip to be positioned in the inferior vena cava when femoral insertion is chosen.

Which site?

There is no right or wrong site for insertion of the double lumen catheter. A number of considerations play a part in site selection. They include the expertise of the clinician, the body habitus of the patient, the presence of other central venous catheters, the presence of a coagulopathy, the presence of intra-abdominal distention and so on.

In most critically ill patients with septic shock and acute renal failure, a pulmonary artery catheter already occupies the right internal jugular or left subclavian veins. The patient is often coagulopathic or thrombocytopenic. The position is often recumbent during much of the day or night. Accordingly, we find the femoral vein an ideal site for insertion. It is typically advised that catheter insertion should be at a point 2–3 cm below and 1 cm medial to the intersection of the femoral pulse and the inguinal ligament. However, we find that at 3 cm below the inguinal ligament, the vein is often mostly behind the artery. Cannulation at this site may result in transection of the femoral artery with the need for surgical repair once the catheter is removed. Accordingly we prefer to cannulate the vein 1 cm below the inguinal ligament. Ultrasound technology is now widely available, however, to help localize the vessel and make catheter insertion much safer[4,5].

Subclavian vein insertion is often considered in patients that are somewhat more mobile. It is important to consider, however, that the subclavian position is most frequently associated with inadequate catheter performance. This phenomenon is due to curving of the catheter under the clavicle, abutting of the catheter tip against the superior vena cava, collapse of the vein against the side or the tip of the catheter in the event of positional changes with decreased central venous pressure and filling. Accordingly, we find the subclavian position generally disappointing and prefer the right jugular vein with a soft catheter that can reach close to, or into, the right atrium to secure adequacy of blood flow rates.

How to care for the site

There are only few controlled studies of catheter site care[6] and none in patients requiring CRRT. In these patients, catheters are often *in situ* for only a week and infection of the catheter is a rare complication. In our unit the incidence of hemofiltration catheter infection is <2%. To protect the site after aseptic catheter insertion with preparation of the skin with chlorhexidine, we use a sandwich technique and a transparent dressing. With this technique an adhesive transparent dressing is placed underneath the catheter and folded into two halves, one half sticks to the skin and the other to the catheter. A second adhesive dressing is placed above the catheter with half of it sticking to the skin and the other half sticking to the catheter and the adhesive dressing below. Thus the 2–3 cm of the catheter closest to the skin are hugged by the two adhesive dressings, which stick to each other's surfaces either side of the catheter entry. This approach makes the catheter dressings less likely to peel off because of sweat and creates a surface that cannot come into contact with contamination from outside. We consider this the ideal way of caring for the insertion site.

Trouble-shooting

Catheters can malfunction or be suspected to harbor infection. If malfunction is suspected, it can be tested for with a syringe containing saline. The venous lumen can be flushed and resistance to flushing can be assessed. Equally, aspirating

through it and assessing resistance to such aspiration of blood can test the 'arterial' limb of the catheter. If resistance is present, it is likely that the catheter limb in question has clotted. Occasionally, however, the problem is positional. This means that, in a given position, the 'arterial' limb cannot function well enough as a channel for blood outflow from the patient but may be adequate for blood inflow. Under such circumstances, the 'venous' limb can be used as the 'arterial' limb and the 'arterial' limb as the 'venous' limb. Switching of the limbs does increase recirculation somewhat, but its practical consequences are usually negligible. In some cases such a switch may be the best way to handle a troublesome access. If such maneuvering fails, or both limbs are dysfunctional, the catheter must be changed. It is then a matter of clinical judgement whether such change is best performed by simple guide wire exchange or whether a new site is needed. The risks and benefits of each approach in a given patient may favor one or the other choice.

If catheter infection is suspected, such infection is often subsequently confirmed in only a minority of patients. Accordingly, the safest approach is to guide wire exchange the catheter and send the tip of the catheter for culture. In most cases such culture will be negative and no further action will be required. If culture of the catheter is positive, then a new catheter will have to be placed at another site and the catheter placed by guide wire exchange will have to be removed. There is no reason to practice regular catheter changes every 4 or 5 days or even more frequently, such an approach is costly, time-consuming and not supported by available information.

References

1. Bellomo R, Parkin G, Love J, Boyce N. A prospective comparative study of continuous arterio-venous hemodiafiltration and continuous veno-venous hemodiafiltration in critically ill patients. *Am J Kidney Dis* 1993; 21: 400–404.
2. Jassal V, Pierratos A. Vascular access for continuous renal replacement therapy. In Ronco C, Bellomo R,

eds. *Critical Care Nephrology*. Dordrecht Kluwer Academic Publishers: 1998; pp 1177–1188.

3. Bellomo R, Ronco C. Circulation of the continuous artificial kidney: blood flow, pressures, clearances and the search for the best. In Ronco C, Artigas A, Bellomo R, eds. *Circulation in Native and Artificial Kidney*. Basel Karger; 1997: pp 138–149.

4. Scott DHT. Editorial. *BJ; Anaesth* 1999; 82: 820–821

5. Hatfield A, Bodenham A. Portable ultrasound for difficult central venous access. *B J Anaesth* 1999; 82: 822–826.

6. Levin A, Mason AJ, Jindall KK, Fong IW, Goldstein MB. Prevention of hemodialysis subclavian vein catheter infection by topical povidone-iodine. *Kidney Int* 1991; 40: 934–938.

17

Nursing Management Concepts for CRRT in the ICU

Ian Baldwin, Tania Elderkin and Nicholas Bridge

Introduction

The introduction of continuous renal replacement therapy in the intensive care unit raises new challenges for the intensive care nurse. Such therapy requires significant nursing infrastructure for it to be successful. Nurses and physicians work closely in this field making it a subspecialty within the intensive care unit. This chapter offers an outline of important steps for the safe and successful nursing management of CRRT in the ICU. Day to day nursing management will be presented as *problem oriented* with the necessary nursing interventions and educational training strategies. Anticoagulant drugs will not be discussed, however, nursing measures to prevent circuit clotting and prolong circuit life are an important nursing consideration and are presented first.

Prevention of circuit clotting

Signs of filter circuit dysfunction or clotting

Obvious clot within the extracorporeal circuit (EC) may necessitate an elective change of some or all components of the EC. Waiting until the circuit clots is undesirable because it usually means that blood cannot easily be returned to the patient. This event leads to the loss of blood and of the entire circuit and filter. Circuits that are packaged as separate components have an advantage over completely prepackaged circuits and filter systems, in that components susceptible to clotting may be changed before the entire system clots. Minimizing patient time off the system when circuits become clotted and reducing cost and waste constitute important economic and environmental advantages of separate component packaging.

The presence of dark streaks through the hollow fibers of filters indicates a degree of filter clotting and perhaps dysfunction but does not necessarily herald imminent filter failure. Filters may perform efficiently and effectively for prolonged periods despite the appearance of such streaking. In *controlled* ultrafiltrate (UF) production systems (pump-off such as using an IV pump), signs of filter failure are less obvious. A possible sign of filter failure is the frequent alarming of the IV (ultrafiltrate) pump. This indicates poor outflow from the filter side of the pump and collapse of the IV line drip chambers due to excessive suction. Measurement of pre- and post-filter pressures or filter gradient may also be useful to determine imminent filter clotting[1] and is a standard feature of modern hemofiltration machines (e.g., Baxter BM 11 & 14, Baxter Health Care, UK).

No anticoagulation
CRRT without anticoagulation is indicated in some patients with intrinsic coagulopathies, e.g. hepatic failure or low platelet counts (<50 000/mm^3). Acceptable filter and circuit life may be achieved without anticoagulation in these patients. Intermittent normal saline flushes have been advocated by some authors but remain unproven in prolonging circuit life[2]. Intermittent flushing does, however, allow the clinician to visualize filter patency and observe for signs of clotting within the EC. The fluid bolus involved may be contraindicated in some patients.

Circuit components relevant to circuit life
Access devices
Access catheter lumen diameter and length play a pivotal role in the ability to adequately allow the passage of blood through the hemofiltration

circuit. Ideally, the access catheter should be large bore, allow access through a single puncture site and provide high flow both to and from the patient during all necessary nursing care activities in the critically ill.

Dual lumen catheters offer significant advantages over single lumen catheters – one entry point and the ability to both draw and return blood via one catheter. Recirculation through the catheter ranges from 5–25%[3,4] and is dependent on internal diameter (ID), catheter length and blood flow rate. Single lumen catheters allow higher flow rates due to greater ID but require two puncture sites.

Access sites
The femoral, internal jugular and subclavian vein are the usual vascular access site for veno-venous systems. Catheters inserted into the thorax may sometimes achieve poor flows due to variation in central filling pressures. This is accentuated by intermittent positive pressure ventilation or the patient sitting upright or out of bed. Intrathoracic catheters, however, allow easier mobilization of the patient, dressing care, and observation of the insertion site. Femoral vein catheters are safer for insertion by a physician but are prone to kinking with hip flexion. Other disadvantages of femoral catheters include decreased patient mobility and difficulty with site dressing.

Blood flow variability at different access sites may also contribute to premature circuit clotting and failure. Unpublished data from research at our institution demonstrated a greater frequency and duration of flow reduction events (delivered blood flow less than that set) at the subclavian site compared with the femoral site. The mean 'life' for filters at the subclavian site was 15.41 hours compared to 25.07 hours at the femoral site. Therefore, the femoral site may be the best for access catheter placement in the critically ill, despite the disadvantages for nursing care, and the site not being easily visible under bed sheets.

Venous bubble trap
Venous air trap/chamber design may be very important to the life of the EC. The air–blood interface within the venous chamber is a potential source of venous chamber clotting and hence

circuit failure. The purpose of this chamber is to prevent any air from the EC entering the patient's circulation. The venous pressure is commonly measured here, and additional IV fluids can be administered through it. Because of this, the level of the blood in the chamber must be below the top to prevent spillage into the pressure transducer line. Most nurses would adjust the blood level to about three-quarters full for visual inspection of blood flow and to ensure air is trapped. Does this air–blood interface promote clotting in the chamber? Data from two studies[5,6] performed at our institution indicate that in excess of 25% of circuit dysfunction occurs primarily as a result of venous chamber clotting. Chamber design incorporating minimal flow stasis and minimal air–blood interface may be a solution to this problem. Blood would therefore enter the chamber below the fluid level in the chamber allowing surface blood to separate forming a plasma layer, which functions as an 'air lock'[7].

Administration of anticoagulants
Anticoagulant drugs such as heparin are best administered via an infusion control device. The administration of anticoagulant drugs via a syringe driver into the circuit means that small volume, high concentration solutions are delivered into the circuit. Administration via a volumetric pump on the other hand, allows the delivery of larger volume, low concentration (dilute) solutions. Syringe drivers are also prone to 'stiction' resulting in variation of instantaneous flow rates[8] and the potential for fluctuations in drug delivery. The delivery of smaller volumes via syringe drivers may result in reduced mixing or streaming of anticoagulant in the blood. The use of high concentration infusions may also predispose to the delivery of little or no anticoagulant into the circuit. The use of a dilute anticoagulant, e.g. heparin 10 IU/ml, and the administration of a higher volume into the circuit may prevent this oscillation in drug delivery, and maximize drug distribution within the EC.

Fluids and fluid management

Continuous therapy in hemofiltration means that large volumes of fluids are required as plasma water replacement or as dialysate. Correspondingly, there are also large volumes of waste. At the clinical level, this problem raises issues with respect to storage and handling; waste disposal; control and monitoring of the fluids; and cost.

Replacement fluids are those used to replace convective plasma water losses. Typically, these fluids are commercially prepared plasma water/electrolyte solutions and are also satisfactory as dialysate for CVVHD, where diffusive clearance is the principal mechanism of solute removal[9]. Such commercially prepared solutions are generally low in potassium (which may have to be added) and may use lactate as a buffer. Lactate is stable in such solutions and is suitable for use in most patients. In critically ill patients who may have difficulty clearing lactate i.e. liver failure, a bicarbonate solution may be necessary. The bicarbonate should be added just prior to use, as it is unstable in solution[9,10,11]. To minimize nursing time, 5 l or larger bags are most appropriate when replacing 1–2 l/h. These fluids are administered at room temperature and thus require warming. A high flow warmer is therefore included in the circuit. Heat loss can occur due to inadequate warming of replacement fluids and compound the heat lost due to the extracorporeal blood circuit itself. Attempts have been made to minimize this by wrapping the lines with aluminum foil or a 'space blanket'[12]. Heat loss, however, may be desirable in some febrile patients. When commercial solutions are not available, a mixture of saline and dextrose solutions (1 l IV bags) is effective as plasma water replacement (see Table 17.1). In this situation, a mixing chamber is useful to mix the solutions 'in line' before administration. The 1 l bags of fluid can be given in rotation if this is not possible. Sterile peritoneal dialysis fluid such as 1.5% Dianeal™ (Baxter Healthcare, Sydney, Australia) can also be used as a dialysate in CVVHD.

Handling and storage of these fluids can be at an 'industrial' level when several patients are being treated concurrently, e.g. one patient treated over a 24 h period with 2 l/h of UF in CVVH (convective clearance) will generate approximately 48 l of waste and require an equivalent volume of plasma water replacement. This means that storage facilities for fluids must be close to the bedside and a large area is needed for the primary supply. Lifting and handling these fluids in these quantities can be an occupational hazard (one 5 l bag weighs approximately 5 kg). To enable gravity flow on the replacement side and the outflow side of the system, bags are often placed at heights, which make handling difficult for nursing staff, i.e. too high or too low. Blood pumps or hemofiltration machines must have a stand or trolley able to support such weight, i.e. 10–20 kg hanging on IV poles as dialysate or replacement, and up to 30 kg of waste. More recent custom-made machines require the solutions to hang under the main blood pump machine as they are weighed automatically, calculating fluid administration/loss and required fluid balance. These trolleys need to be sturdy and well balanced to facilitate movement around the beside without toppling over. In a *spontaneous* or *IV pump off* effluent system, discussed below, the filtrate can be placed on the floor. These practical problems in addition to the cost of commercial solutions have led some investigators to explore the on-line production of replacement fluids[13].

Control and monitoring of fluids incorporating waste disposal

The removal and replacement of fluids in CVVH or CVVHD is often set to produce a fluid loss but occasionally the system may be managed to yield no loss, i.e. a 'zero' balance. Therefore, IV fluids and drugs administered via central venous lines and/or pulmonary artery catheters are independent of the replacement fluids given in the system. These fluids, however, should be

Table 17.1: Plasma water replacement regimen for continuous hemofiltration. Litre bags given in rotation or mixed evenly via a multi connector and mixing chamber. (Modified and reproduced from the *Australian and New Zealand Journal of Medicine*, Vol. 20, 1990).

Litre no.	Constitution	Additives
1	N saline.	nil
2	N saline.	10 ml 10% Ca gluconate
3	N saline.	5 mM $MgSO_4$
4	5% dextrose	150 ml 8.4% $NaHCO_3$

taken into account when prescribing the hourly fluid balance required for a 24-hour period.

Ultrafiltrate generation controlled by mini roller pumps can be integrated into the machine fluid balance system by using scales to assess movement of fluid by weight. The filtrate generated in spontaneous or pump-off method requires disposal. Collection techniques vary amongst clinical areas, however, with IV pump or mini roller pump generation a sealed system where large volumes are collected before disposal is common. Large plastic bags with 25–30 l capacity can be used with the filtrate line discharging directly into a sealed opening. Empty or used plasma water replacement bags can be used to collect the filtrate. This system embraces a bag recycling process. However, only 5 l can be directed to a single bag (the volume of the replacement fluid bag when full). Several bags can be used in parallel using a multiport connector. This system allows larger volumes to be collected before bag changes. Direct drainage or collection into a 20 l bucket is also performed in some institutions with the IV pump method. Direct discharge into a sewage outlet reduces nursing time, but requires a non-weigh method of fluid measurement, i.e. an IV pump and a suitable outlet next to the bed area.

In order to maintain satisfactory fluid balance, a hemofiltration system needs to have accurate control of the fluids and be integrated into the blood pump operation. The IV pump system has the disadvantage that the blood pump does not communicate with the IV pumps to cease fluid removal when blood flow is interrupted. If filtration continues when there is little or no blood flow, the hematocrit may increase enough to cause clotting in the hemofilter. The nurse must manually pause the IV pumps quickly when the blood flow stops and then restart filtration after blood flow recommences. There is no such hazard with the inflow or replacement IV pumps/fluids. The volume of filtrate generation is also limited, as most standard IV pumps are limited at 1 l per hour. Two pumps in parallel or a dual channel pump would be required for a 2 l per hour ultrafiltrate. Weigh scale systems are potentially highly accurate and may be the only safe method in the pediatric setting. In 'IV pump off', a fluid balance error on the filtrate side of

the circuit can be anticipated. This error is dependent on the pump's operating specifications and upon the type of therapy. During CVVHD, where the dialysate solution is above the filter and flowing past the blood in the membrane, the IV pumps have a steady head of pressure driving them on the effluent side and fluid balance errors should be decreased. In CVVH, with convective clearance, however, negative pressure arises in the filtrate line as the IV pumps suck on the membrane to generate plasma water effluent. This suction is likely to induce greater fluid balance inaccuracy. These inaccuracies are also influenced by the membrane size or surface area and blood pump speed. In a $0.75 m^2$ AN 69® F 8 (Hospal, Lyon, France) filter with a blood flow of 200 ml/min, and the IV pump set at 2 l/h, the pressure in the effluent line will be positive for approximately 3.5 h of a new filter's life[14]. During this time, the membrane is providing more effluent than the pump set rate. After this, as protein and cell deposition occurs in the membrane, the effluent line pressure becomes negative and the IV pump 'sucks' on the membrane. It is at this time that the IV pump may become more inaccurate and thus approach the limits of its specifications. Many IV pumps have a specified operating error of up to ±5% of set rate. At an effluent rate of 2 l/h, a 5% error would be 100 ml per hour or a possible 2.4 l effluent error over 24 hours. In a study using an IV GEMINI PC2® (IMED, San Diego, USA) the measured error was consistently in the positive but within 3% of set rate, i.e. more effluent was generated than displayed on the pump digital readout[14]. These findings are consistent with those of others[15] who employed this pump in the CAVHD mode. Furthermore, Roberts and colleagues[16] also found that, during *in vitro* CVVHD, the outflow pump delivered 3.6% more than the set rate. Weighing the UF after a set time interval (1–4 hours) using simple kitchen scales can reduce the fluid loss calculation error. The collection bag weight is deducted from the gross weight when the waste bag is changed and weighed. The weight in grams equals the volume in ml. Fluids replacement can also be weighed but as the IV pumps are operating in a conventional manner, the digital display is more accurate[14].

Therefore, a system for continuous renal replacement therapies, with IV pumps in conjunction with a basic blood pump is generally considered reliable and acceptable for clinical use in adult patients. A summary of the advantages and disadvantages for each method is provided in Table 17.2. The fluid balance management required in CVVH(D) has been described as a 'potential nightmare'[12] due to the large volumes involved. Despite the potential fluid balance error when using IV pump off, we consider it a simple, efficient, safe, reliable and low cost system in the adult patient.

Nursing management of patients undergoing CRRT

Nursing management of the patient undergoing CVVH incorporates many aspects of general management of critically ill patients: psychological care, care of the immobilized patient, and family involvement. Specific aspects of nursing management related to CVVH are outlined below.

With any health care technology, it is easy to focus on management of the machinery involved and lose sight of the patient[17]. It is therefore valuable to use a *problem-oriented* approach to care, although checklists such as the Trouble-shooting Guide (Table 17.3) can be very useful for novice practitioners. Much of the patient management described below can also be applied to patients undergoing other forms of CRRT.

Problem oriented patient management – nursing interventions

Potential fluid and electrolyte imbalance
Related to high volume filtrate removal and fluid replacement.

Monitoring of patient fluid status
Status is monitored via physical assessment and hemodynamic parameters.

Assessing fluid balance
The fluid balance chart is essential for assessment of the patient's fluid status and for the prescription of correct fluid therapy. When using an IV pump system and *prospective* fluid management as

---

Table 17.2: Summary advantages and disadvantages of IV pump generated ultrafiltrate combined with a simple blood pump *versus* mini roller pumps found in purpose built hemofiltration machines.

	IV pumps generating ultrafiltrate connected to a bag or bottle	Mini roller pumps generating ultrafiltrate with an automatic scale weigh system
Cost	Low. (Flexibility to use IV pumps for other uses.)	High. As part of custom made machines.*,**
Fluid balance calculation	Manual readings from the IV pumps for replacement and ultrafiltrate hourly, or weigh fluids at 1–4 hours.	Automatic integration for hourly and desired net daily fluid loss.*,**
Accuracy	Within that of the IV pumps specifications (e.g. ± 5%).	Accurate according to manufacturers.
Collection and disposal	Discharge into a bag or bottle. Direct discharge into sluice possible.	Bags only, due to weigh system. No direct discharge possible.
Integration into blood pump function	No. Require a manual step to pause pumps if blood pump stops or ↑ risk of clotting in filter.	Yes. Both ultrafiltrate and replacement mini roller pumps stop together when the blood pump stops.
Rate max per hour	Limited to 1 litre per hour. Twin channel pumps or multiple pumps in parallel to 2–4–6 litres/hour.	Up to 11 litres per hour.*

* Baxter BM 11 & 14 (Baxter Health Care, U.K). ** Baxter BM 11 & 14 & Prisma (CGH Medical, USA).

previously described, hourly calculation of CVVH input/output is common. This can be charted as in the example shown in Table 17.4. With

integrated systems, e.g. Prisma (CGH Medical, USA) only the net fluid loss from the CVVH is recorded hourly. Some authors advocate using a

Table 17.3: CVVH troubleshooting guide

Alarm/problem	possible causes	Nursing actions
Low blood outflow e.g. low arterial pressure alarm	a. Kinked or clamped outflow line b. Inadequate blood flow from access device due to: Clotted access device or outflow line of circuit Kinking of access device Patient position Access device against vessel wall Hypovolemia/hypotension	a. Remove obstruction. b. Check/declot access device. Reposition patient. Change clotted outflow line. Consider swapping outflow line to other lumen of access device Consult medical staff *re* hypotension, or access device placement
Low blood flow in return line e.g. low venous pressure alarm	a. Line separation or disconnection in circuit b. Circuit kinked or clamped between hemofilter and return-flow pressure alarm c. Clotted hemofilter d. Blood pump speed too slow or alarm limit set too low e. Isolator sensor line dysfunction (eg. collapsed, disconnected)	a. Check lines, discard if disconnection has occurred b. Remove obstruction c. Change hemofilter, reassess anticoagulation d. Correct pump speed or alarm setting e. Change isolator
High pressure in blood return line e.g. high venous pressure alarm	a. Clotted return line, b. Circuit kinked or clamped between return-flow pressure alarm and access c. Clot in access device d. Change in patient position e. Isolator sensor line dysfunction (e.g. clamped, blood clot in)	a. Change return line and other circuit components as necessary. Reassess anticoagulation b. Remove obstruction c. De-clot access device. Reassess anticoagulation d. Reposition patient e. Change/un-clamp isolator
Air detected in blood return line e.g. air detection alarm	a. Line separation or disconnection b. Air detection chamber incorrectly positioned, or blood level too low in chamber c. Frothing or turbulence in chamber	a. Check lines, discard if disconnection has occurred b. Reposition chamber, or raise blood level c. Remove excess froth with syringe, if unsuccessful change air detection chamber (NB: if large amounts of air are present, disconnect and discard entire blood circuit).
Low UF flow e.g. Ultrafiltrate pump alarms 'obstruction-fluid side'	a. Clotted hemofilter b. Kinked or clamped ultrafiltrate line	a. Change hemofilter. Reassess anticoagulation b. Remove obstruction c. Check pump speed adequate

NB: Any delay in trouble-shooting the CVVH system will increase the risk of circuit clotting – the blood pump should be off for no longer than 3–5 minutes. If using IV infusion pumps for replacement fluid and UF control, pause pumps if blood flow is not re-established within approx. 30 seconds. New machines avoide this as pumps are integrated to stop together.

Table 17.4: Fluid balance chart for: U.F. @ 2 l/h and replacement @ 1765/h. Total IN = replacement + heparin First hour 1765 + 35 = 1800. Desired hourly loss −200 ml

HF anticoagulation (heparin)	Replacement fluids IN	Total INPUT	Ultrafiltrate OUT	Hourly balance	Total progressive balance
35	1765	1800	2000	−200	−200
35	1750	1785	2000	−215	−415
35	1755	1790	2000	−210	−625
35	1743	1778	2025	−247	−872
35	etc.				

Note: The IV pump (in or out) volumes will vary according to the exact time they are checked, i.e. they are not integrated together. Weighing U.F. using simple scales can reduce errors in fluid removal calculations.

specific CVVH chart to document the inflow/outflow[18], however, it may be more useful to include the CVVH data on the general fluid balance chart. This allows staff to interpret the patient's *total* fluid balance more easily.

Maintaining CVVH input and output
With high volume filtration and fluid replacement, it is important that blood flow rates be maintained. In non-integrated systems even brief interruptions to either filtration or replacement can result in significant changes to the net fluid balance[19]. If technical difficulties are encountered with replacement, for example, filtration rate should be adjusted to prevent large fluid losses. In integrated systems such as the Prisma (CGH Medical, USA), the replacement and ultrafiltrate pumps are programmed to stop together so that fluid imbalance is not such a problem.

Monitoring serum electrolytes
Recommendations for the frequency of laboratory samples vary greatly[20]. Frequent monitoring may be necessary initially, whereas the 'stable' CVVH patient may only require serum analysis twice daily.

Potential for poor clearance of waste/excess fluid
Related to deterioration in filter function or a non-continuous system.

Maintaining blood flow through the filter
The blood flow should ideally be maintained at around 200 ml/min. At times, this may not be possible due to the patient's cardiovascular status or poor vascular access. In these situations flow should always be maintained at >100 ml/min[19]. Rapid trouble-shooting is important to prevent prolonged cessation or slowing of blood flow.

Clotting
Clotting in the filter has been identified as a major problem in filter function[21,22]. Nursing interventions to minimize coagulation in the extracorporeal circuit include:

Maintaining pre-dilution
Administration of replacement fluids before the filter may prolong filter function[23]. Rapid trouble-shooting is again important to prevent slowing or cessation of replacement fluid infusion.

Maintaining anticoagulation
Anticoagulation will be ordered according to patient status and physician preference. It must be maintained at the appropriate rate and the patient monitored carefully. As previously noted, running infusions at very slow rates (i.e <5 ml/h) has been shown to lead to variability in flow rates[8] and increases the potential for low, or no, anticoagulant delivery. The use of very dilute heparin (e.g. 10 IU/ml) at a greater rate will help to minimize this problem and may improve the efficacy of anticoagulation effect[23].

Correct priming technique
When priming a new CRRT circuit it is important to minimize residual air bubbles and preservative

agents such as glycerine, as these may increase clotting in the filter. The use of circuits pre-primed by the manufacturer may be of benefit.

Monitoring for early signs of filter clotting
This includes monitoring the circuit for the signs of circuit dysfunction as previously noted. Flushing the circuit with normal saline once per shift or when clotting is suspected may allow visual detection of clotting in the filter.

Maintaining a continuous system
It is important for CRRT to operate continuously to maintain clearance of solutes. If the circuit has to be disconnected, or the filtration stopped for any reason, it should be recommenced as soon as possible, particularly in highly atozemic patients.

Potential for infection
Related to invasive procedure/access device.

Maintaining asepsis during all procedures
This includes priming, connection and disconnection of the circuit, changing fluid flasks and dressing the access device. **Regular changing of flush flasks**: at least every 48 hours. **Monitoring patient**: signs of local or systemic infection should be detected early. CRRT may mask fever due to its cooling effect (heat loss via the extracorporeal circuit).

Potential infection risk to others
Related to extracorporeal blood circuit.

Follow infection control guidelines at all times
Take extra care with disposal of used circuits and avoiding the use of needles to sample blood from the circuit.

Potential blood loss
Potential blood loss related to clotting of circuit, circuit disconnection/leak, rupture of filter fibers or anticoagulation-related hemorrhage.

Minimizing blood loss
This can be accomplished by: a) returning circuit blood to patient whenever possible, i.e. before circuit clots completely; b) maintaining patency of circuit by ensuring connections are luer locked

and visible and by setting appropriate alarms to detect early leaks (e.g. low venous pressure); c) monitoring filtrate for color changes indicating fibre rupture (some CRRT machines have blood leak detectors on the filtrate line); d) monitoring for signs of excess anticoagulation. Bleeding has been shown to be a potential complication during CRRT[24], it is therefore important to minimize anticoagulation where possible and to detect any early signs by testing gastric aspirate and urine (if any) for blood, monitoring neurological status, vital signs and laboratory measures of clotting.

Potential heat loss
Related to high volume fluid replacement and extracorporeal circuit.

Warming replacement fluid
A high volume fluids warmer should be used and is most important for heating the dialysate in CVVHD(F) mode. **Monitoring patient's temperature, warming patient**: insulating or warming blankets may be used. **Insulating the circuit**: this technique has not been proven to be of specific benefit in preventing hypothermia in CRRT and could increase heat loss due to surface heat radiation if aluminum foil is used without a further covering layer of plastic or papercloth. Such insulation will prevent easy visual monitoring of the circuit.

Immobility
Related to procedure/access device.

ICU policies may vary on this issue
Generally, bedrest is maintained for patients with femoral access devices. Patients with subclavian or jugular access devices are able to sit out of bed if their general condition permits. In some cases, the circuit can be disconnected to allow a patient to ambulate. This must be assessed as a significant benefit to the patient given the work/hazards involved. Stopping the blood pump and system momentarily is best during sitting a patient out of bed.

Potential reactions to foreign substances
Related to circuit components and sterilizing agents.

Using highly biocompatible circuit components[23].
Flushing the filter
At least 1 l of normal saline should be flushed
through the filter *immediately* prior to use.

Other day to day management issues

In order for CVVH to run smoothly, it is
important to have clear, written protocols, and
guidelines for procedures and management,
particularly in the following areas: a) priming
technique; b) connection and disconnection
procedures; c) maintaining patent circuits after
procedure related disconnection; d) medical
guidelines for the patient regarding level of
anticoagulation, fluid balance and indications for
alternative renal therapies.

Staff expertise
The introduction of any new technology into an
ICU creates the need for education and clinical
support to ensure safety and efficiency of patient
care[20]. Some authors suggest that, when
introducing CRRT to critical care nurses, little or
no specialized training is required[21,25,26]. In
order to manage this therapy at a high standard,
however, a significant educational program is
mandatory. New developments in the therapy and
high staff turnover mandate that the program
must be ongoing and continuous.

The education program should allow staff to
enter an expertise pathway with three levels
comparable to Benner's[27] application of the
Dreyfus and Dreyfus model of skill acquisition in
nursing: novice/advanced beginner, competent,
proficient/expert (Table 17.5). In order to attain
adequate staff expertise Talbot *et al.*[28] describe a
staged education program utilizing a complex
patient simulator. Although this may not be
practical in some settings, a simple simulator can
be created using a resuscitation doll connected to
a CRRT system with food dye instilled into the
saline filled circuit. An access catheter can be
placed into a saline bag in the groin of the doll
and the system set to function. This set up is
cheap, very practical and a useful teaching tool
(Figure 17.1). Each ICU needs to set up a
program to meet its specific needs utilizing the
resources available. The education program
should be multi-faceted, to create interest in the
subject matter, and to cater for individual needs
and learning styles. Some suggested approaches
are outlined below.

Inservice sessions
Didactic lectures may be useful to introduce the
basic concepts of CRRT; however, adult learners,
such as critical care nurses, respond better to
discussion groups and practical sessions.
Knowledge of the CRRT circuit can easily be

Table 17.5: Staff expertise in CRRT.

Expertise level	Skill level
Novice/advanced beginner	Basic nursing care of the CRRT patient
	Monitoring of the CRRT system
	Identify major problems in the system
	Require clinical support for priming and trouble-shooting
Competent	**Mastery of the above**
	Using written guidelines for reference be able to:
	Set-up and prime system
	Initiate and cease CRRT (including connection/disconnection procedures)
	Trouble-shoot alarms and anticipate problems
Proficient/expert	**Mastery of the above**
	Modifying circuits: convert from CVVH to CVVHDF
	Advanced trouble-shooting
	Management of anticoagulation regimes
	Teach others
	Protocol development
	Liaison with biomedical suppliers

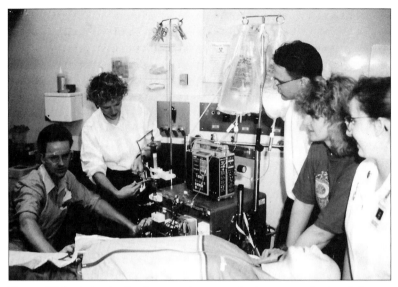

Figure 17.1: A simple simulator can be created using a resuscitation doll connected to a CRRT system with food dye instilled into the saline filled circuit. An access catheter can be placed into a saline bag in the groin of the doll and the system set to function.

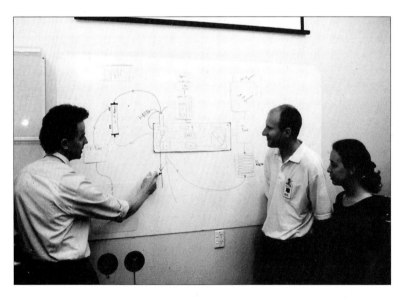

Figure 17.2: Cardboard cut-outs of system components asking the learners to 'put the circuit together' by sticking them onto a writing board and drawing in the blood/replacement/filtrate lines.

addressed by using cardboard cut-outs of system components and getting the participants to 'put the circuit together' by sticking them onto a writing board and drawing in the blood/replacement/filtrate lines (Figure 17.2).

They can then discuss and identify common faults and alarm problems. Sessions covering priming circuits, connection/disconnection to the patient, and trouble-shooting should include both demonstration and guided practice at the bedside.

Reference material and study guides

Although time consuming to produce, resource materials such as Woodrow's[29] hemofiltration package, can be very valuable for part-time, weekend and night-duty staff, whose access to other educational resources may be limited. Reference material can also include clear written protocols, guidelines and checklists to assist novice practitioners and provide backup for more experienced staff.

Seminars

Two or three day seminars that include both theoretical and practical aspects of CRRT are an excellent way to educate a large number of staff. The availability of circuits/simulator for mock set-up/trouble-shooting allows the nurse to practice new skills in a non-stressful environment. Individual clinical instruction although time consuming, can be an invaluable part of an education program. It allows the nurse to reinforce and clarify learning from seminars, study guides, and inservice sessions and also provides the educators with feedback on the adequacy of the education program and the expertise of each individual.

Generally, staff will learn the basics of CRRT from an education program, but eventually only gain real expertise from practice when the system is functioning on a patient in their care. Regular follow up of learning with bedside instruction provides consolidation for the learner and feedback to the teacher (Figure 17.3). Consolidation of learning is therefore dependent on the frequency of CRRT use in the patient population[28]. This creates a slower learning curve than in dialysis units where experience can be gained more readily.

In any ICU, it is desirable to have a majority of staff functioning at the 'competent' level, with small groups of staff at the 'novice' and 'expert' levels. Unfortunately, reality often sees great fluctuations in the expertise levels available. The charge nurse/clinical supervising nurse should therefore review staffing for this skill mix on a regular basis, not only for daily staffing but also in the overall staffing of the unit. The continuous nature of this therapy demands that staff across a 24 hour period have the required expertise.

In addition to a comprehensive education program, there are some other ways to improve staff expertise and standards of care: a) allocate 'novice' practitioners to care for patients on CRRT. A 'competent or expert' support person should be allocated to an adjacent patient, available to assist them. This practical exposure stimulates interest, relieves anxieties and promotes confidence. b) Encourage the

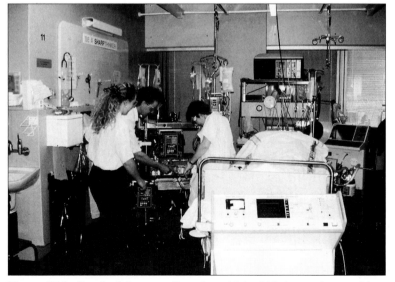

Figure 17.3: Regular follow up of learning with bedside instruction provides consolidation for the learner and feedback to the teacher.

'competent and expert' nurses to run clinical in service sessions to improve their confidence and knowledge and provide role models for the 'novice' practitioners. c) Undertake quality assurance (QA). Evaluation of the care of patients undergoing CRRT will identify problem areas and encourage improvement in standards. Kaplow and Bendo[30] described the application of a unit-based QA tool specifically related to CAVH, focusing on problem areas such as fluid balance monitoring. This tool could easily be adapted to CVVH. Multi-disciplinary approaches to QA are also beneficial[31], particularly in areas such as anticoagulation management. Any data collection will create discussion and thought, which aids development of clinical skills.

Conclusion

In conclusion, the effective and safe nursing management of CRRT in the intensive care unit requires a detailed understanding of the principles of therapy, the determinants of circuit life, and the importance of accurate fluid balancing. Such management can therefore be achieved only in an environment which incorporates clear protocols, continuing theoretical education, and frequent supervised practical use of techniques. In such an environment, CRRT is easily incorporated into the therapies available in the ICU and operates smoothly and safely to offer the patient a modern and highly effective organ support therapy.

References

1. Bierer P, Holt AW. Continuous venovenous haemodiafiltration: Monitoring circuit function. *Blood Purif* 1995; 13: 385–402.

2. Ward D, Mehta R. Extracorporeal management of acute renal failure patients at high risk of bleeding. *Kidney Int* 1993; 43(S41): S237–244.

3. Dembitsky W. Adult placenta. Vascular access for peripheral organ support. *ASAIO J* 1996; 42: 12–15.

4. Macias WL, Clark WR. Azotemia control by extracorporeal therapy in patients with acute renal failure. *New Horiz* 1995; 4: 688–698.

5. Baldwin I, Bridge N, Heland M *et al.* The effect of heparin administration site on extracorporeal circuit life during continuous venovenous hemofiltration. *Aust Crit Care* 1996; 1: 29.

6. Baldwin I, Bridge N, Heland M *et al.* The effect of filter configuration on extracorporeal circuit life during continuous veno-venous haemofiltration. *Aust Crit Care* 1996; 9: 22.

7. Gretz N, Quintel M, Ragaller M *et al.* Low-dose heparinization for anticoagulation in intensive care patients on continuous hemofiltration. *Contrib Nephro* 1995; 116: 130–135.

8. Stull J, Erenberg A, Leff R. Flow rate variability from electronic infusion devices. *Crit Care Med* 1988; 16: 888–891.

9. Ronco C, Barbacini S, Digito A, Zoccali G. Achievements and new directions in continuous renal replacement therapies. *New Horiz* 1995; 3: 708–716.

10. Clasen M, Bohm R, Riehl J *et al.* Lactate or bicarbonate for intermittent haemofiltration. *Contrib Nephrol* 1991; 93: 152–155.

11. DeLuca PP, Kowalsky RJ. Problems arising from the transfer of sodium bicarbonate injection from ampoules to plastic disposable syringes. *Am J Hosp Pharm* 1972; 29: 217–222.

12. Miller R, Kingswood C, Bullen C, Cohen S. Renal replacement therapy in the ICU: the role of continuous arteriovenous haemodialysis. *Br J Hosp Med* 1990; 43: 354–362.

13. Canaud B, Flavier JL, Argiles A *et al.* Hemodiafiltration with on-line production of substitution fluid: Long-term safety and quantitative assessment of efficacy. *Contrib Nephrol* 1994; 108: 12–22.

14. Baldwin I, Bridge N, Merrony N *et al.* IV pump-controlled ultrafiltrate in CVVH: digital values versus measured volume and relationship to ultrafiltrate pressure. *Aust Crit Care* 1996; 9: 22–23.

15. Bosworth C, Swann S, Paganini E. Evaluation of the IMED Gemini PC2 volumetric infusion pumps in extracorporeal continuous therapy circuits. *Dialysis and Transplantation* 1990; 19: 126–128.

16. Roberts M, Winney RJ. Errors in fluid balance with pump control of continuous hemodialysis. *Int J Artif Organs* 1992; 15: 99–102.

17. Sinclair V. High technology in critical care: implications for nursing's role and practice. *Focus Crit Care* 1988; 15: 36–41.

18. Lievaart A, Voerman HJ. Nursing management of continuous arteriovenous hemodialysis. *Heart Lung* 1991; 20: 152–158.

19. Kox WJ, Rohr U, Wauer H. Practical aspects of renal replacement therapy. *Int J Artif Organs* 1996; 19: 100–105.

20. Palmer JC, Koorejian K, London JB, Dechert RE, Bartlett RH. Nursing management of continuous arteriovenous hemofiltration for acute renal failure. *Focus Crit Care* 1986; 13: 21–30.

21. Price C. Continuous arteriovenous ultrafiltration: A monitoring guide for ICU nurses. *Crit Care Nurse* 1989; 9: 12–19.

22. Coloski D, Mastrianni J, Dube R, Brown LH. Continuous arteriovenous hemofiltration patient: Nursing care plan. *Dimens Crit Care Nurse* 1990; 9: 130–142.

23. Golper TA, Price J. Continuous venovenous hemofiltration for acute renal failure in the intensive care setting. *ASAIO J* 1994; 40: 936–939.

24. Sigler M, Manns M. CRRT in the critically ill patient with acute renal failure. *ASAIO J* 1994; 40: 928–930.

25. Winkleman C. Hemofiltration: A new technique in critical care nursing. *Heart Lung* 1985; 14: 265–271.

26. Dirkes S. How to use the new CVVH renal replacement systems. *Am J Nurse* 1994; May: 67–73.

27. Benner P. *The Dreyfus Model of Skill Acquisition Applied to Nursing. From Novice to Expert. Excellence and Power in Clinical Nursing Practice.* California: Addison Wesley Pub. Co. 1984: 13–38.

28. Talbot TL, Rosenthal CH, Strider VC. Collaborative development of a patient simulator for educating nurses in hemofiltration therapies. *Biomed Instrum Technol* 1994; 28: 271–281.

29. Woodrow P. Resource package: haemofiltration. *Intens Crit Care Nurse* 1993; 9: 95–107.

30. Kaplow R, Bendo K. QA in continuous arteriovenous hemofiltration. *Dimens Crit Care Nurse* 1989; 8: 170–174 .

31. Baldwin I, Elderkin T. Continuous hemofiltration: Nursing perspectives in critical care. *New Horiz* 1995; 3: 738–747.

18

Drug Dosing Adjustments During Continuous Renal Replacement Therapies

Thomas Golper

Introduction

This review will focus on how to make drug dosing adjustments for CRRT based on known pharmacokinetic and solute removal principles (see Chapter 3, Solute Transport).

Total body drug clearance is the sum of 'regional' clearances, which may include hepatic, renal, other body metabolic pathways or extracorporeal devices. For a regional clearance to be considered clinically significant it must exceed 30% of total body clearance. Drugs significantly removed by glomerular filtration are most affected by CRRTs. A drug under normal circumstances with a renal clearance that constitutes >30% of total body clearance is likely to experience substantial removal during CRRT and will require dosing supplementation. Other major drug properties that affect clearance by CRRT include protein binding (PB) and volume of distribution (V_d). Molecular weight, drug charge, water or lipid solubility, and membrane binding are minor factors.

Major drug properties affecting removal by CRRT

The **volume of distribution** (V_d) of a drug is a manifestation of its tissue binding, a mathematical construct that presumes a volume as if all the drug in the body is distributed equally into a homogeneous reservoir at the concentration noted in blood. A large V_d (arbitrarily defined as >0.6 l/ kg, the total body water space) reflects a drug that is highly tissue bound and not particularly accessible to the circulation. Such drugs are unlikely to be delivered to the CRRT sufficiently to result in clinically significant

removal and supplemental dosing may not be necessary.

The drug's **protein binding (PB)**, especially to albumin, is another major drug property affecting CRRT elimination. Only free or unbound drug is available for pharmacologic action, metabolism, excretion, and removal by CRRT. The molecular weight of the unbound drug and its V_d impact the drug's removal by CRRT. A solute with a small V_d which is 30% unbound probably demonstrates rapid equilibration with the circulation. Hence, its removal by CRRT may be substantial. Alternatively, the CRRT removal of a drug which is 50% unbound but has a large V_d will be much more influenced by the V_d than by the reasonably large unbound fraction. The sieving coefficient (ratio of the filtrate concentration to that in the plasma retentate) of 60 drugs measured during continuous hemofiltration correlates well ($r = 0.74$, $P < 0.001$) with the known unbound fraction (Table 18.1).

Factors which alter drug binding to circulating proteins include pH, hyperbilirubinemia, displacement by other drugs, heparin, free fatty acids and the molar ratios of drug to protein. These phenomena, as well as the minor drug properties discussed below, probably explain the slight discrepancies noted between the sieving coefficient and the unbound fraction (Table 18.1).

Minor drug properties affecting removal by CRRT

Drug charge affects clearance by the Gibbs–Donnan effect created by retained anionic proteins (e.g. albumin) on the blood side of the

Table 18.1: Drug sieving coefficients during hemofiltration.

Sieving coefficients	Observed	Expected*
Antibiotics		
Amikacin	0.95	0.95
Amphotericin B	0.35	0.10
Ampicillin	0.69	0.80
Cefmenoxime	0.54	0.58
Cefoperazone	0.27	0.10
Cefotaxime	1.06	0.62
Cefotiam	0.95	0.60
Cefoxitin	0.83	0.59
Ceftazidime	0.90	0.83
Ceftriaxone	0.20	0.15
Cephapirin	1.48	0.55
Cilastatin	0.75	0.56
Ciprofloxacin	0.58	0.60
Clindamycin	0.49	0.40
Doxycycline	0.40	0.20
Erythromycin	0.37	0.30
Fluconazole	1.00	0.88
Flucytosine	0.80	0.90
Gentamicin	0.81	0.95
Imipenem	0.90	0.80
Metronidazole	0.84	0.80
Mezlocillin	0.71	0.68
Nafcillin	0.55	0.20
Netilmicin	0.93	0.95
Oxacillin	0.02	0.05
Perfloxacin	0.80	0.80
Pencillin	0.68	0.50
Piperacillin	0.82	0.80
Streptomycin	0.30	0.65
Sulfamethoxazole	0.30	0.60
Teichoplanin	0.05	0.10
Tobramycin	0.90	0.95
Vancomycin	0.80	0.90
Miscellaneous		
Amrinone	0.80	0.70
Bromide	1.00	1.00
Chlordiazepoxide	0.05	0.05
Cisplatin	0.10	0.10
Clofibrate	0.06	0.04
Cyclosporine	0.58	0.10
Diathybarbital	1.00	0.90
Diazepam	0.02	0.02
Digoxin	0.70	0.80
Digitoxin	0.15	0.05
Famotidine	0.73	0.85
Glyburide	0.60	0.01
Glutethimide	0.02	0.50
Lidocaine	0.14	0.36
Lithium	0.90	1.00
Metamizole	0.40	0.40
N-acetyl procainamide	0.92	0.90
Nizatidine	0.59	0.65
Nitrazepam	0.08	0.10
Nomifensin	0.70	0.40
Oxazepam	0.10	0.10
Phenobarbital	0.80	0.60
Phenytoin	0.45	0.10
Phosphomycin	0.24	0.90
Procainamide	0.86	0.86
Ranitidine	0.78	0.85
Theophylline	0.80	0.47

* The expected coefficient assumes that protein binding is the sole determinant of drug sieving and that protein binding is as stated in the Bennett Tables (see text), i.e. in healthy subjects. Observed coefficients correlate with expected coefficients with r = 0.74 and $P < 0.001$.

membrane. Some drugs (e.g. aminoglycosides) avidly **bind to certain membranes** (e.g. AN69) such that the drug is removed from the circulation but is not detected in the dialysate/filtrate[6]. Some time later it may be displaced from the membrane. Large surface area AN69 membranes may permanently bind >20 mg of aminoglycosides. The significance will depend on the size of the dose. **Molecular weight** (MW) had been an important theoretical determinant of removal by CRRT, but as the membranes and techniques increase efficiency, drug MW becomes a less important factor. Larger MW has more of a retarding influence on diffusive transport than it does during convective transport, but the diffusion through high flux membranes has made this difference much smaller. Larger MW drugs require more time for diffusion but with blood pumping, more blood is processed per unit of time and with CRRTs more time is available, again rendering MW a less important determinant of elimination Also, blood pumping increases the transmembrane pressure, generating a significant component of convective removal, which enhances the transport of larger molecular weight solutes. Thus, while MW is of theoretical importance, drug removal by CRRT is actually not dependent on it because most drugs are <1500 daltons.

Hemodialyzer/filter properties which affect drug removal

In CRRT effective **solute pore size** parallels **hydraulic permeability** (low pressure ultrafiltration potential/surface area). Essentially, membranes that are porous to water are also porous to unbound drugs. Membrane **surface area** is important and directly correlated for both convective and diffusive transport. This becomes particularly relevant to removal of solute by adsorption to the membrane.

CRRT operational conditions that affect drug removal

Continuous hemofiltration operating by spontaneous blood flow will generate ultrafiltration rates (UFR) of 10–16 ml/min, equivalent to a GFR of 10–16. Using a blood pump with Q_b of 125 to 250 ml/min, UFR increase to 20–30 ml/min. Thus, during continuous hemofiltration, depending on the specific operating conditions, a clearance comparable to a GFR of 10–30 ml/min can be achieved. If continuous dialysis is used, there is still a component of convection applied, generally a UFR of 1 to 10 ml/min. The dialytic contribution to clearance is 15–20 ml/min, based on the dialysate flow rate (Q_d). Most CRRTs apply high flux membranes and Q_d of 16 to 34 ml/min. Therefore, continuous dialysis and hemofiltration provide similar clearances. Regarding drug dosing recommendations, it is helpful to think of the CRRT as a GFR of 10–50 ml/min, especially when using drug dosing references which utilize GFR levels in the recommendations (see Aronoff GR *et al. Drug Prescribing in Renal Failure: Dosing Guidelines for Adults.* 4th edition. American College of Physicians, Philadelphia, 1998).

Estimating drug removal by CRRT

Quantifying drug removal is helpful to estimate supplemental dosing. The easiest way is to utilize the Bennett Tables. Using urea clearance as a reference point, a standard hemodialysis provides a urea clearance of 180 ml/min for 4 hours. Since CRRT in a day runs 6 times as long, 1/6th of the clearance is needed (30 ml/min) for a day of CRRT treatment to provide approximately the same daily dose of dialysis as a standard treatment. Thus, if one has experience with a particular drug in patients receiving regular hemodialysis and

specific information is unavailable for CRRT, a simple extrapolation will suffice. Aggressive CRRT is equivalent to daily hemodialysis.

For pure convective therapies determination of drug removal is straightforward. The unbound fraction is filtered (Table 18.1). The drug concentration in the filtrate will be the plasma concentration times the unbound fraction. Plasma levels have peaks and troughs, but for drugs following first order kinetics, as do most drugs, the steady state level (C_{ss}) is the mean of the peak and trough. The easiest way to estimate the quantity removed by convective CRRT is to assume that the C_{ss} represents the average level. The filtrate concentration is the C_{ss} times the unbound fraction. The total quantity removed (and presumably the amount one desires to replace) is the filtrate concentration times the filtrate volume. Thus, a C_{ss} can be valuable in estimating losses and supplemental doses. Mathematically, this can be summarized as the following equation:

Equation 1   Supplemental dose = $C_{ss} \times$ unbound fraction $\times$ UFR $\times$ Dosing interval.

Drug dosing recommendations during CRRT

There are four approaches to specific recommendations for drug dosing during CRRT. The first and strongly suggested approach is to utilize the Bennett Tables. This is helpful for the agents in most frequent use that are included in the tables.

Another approach is to apply the principles discussed here to estimate supplements based on losses. But this results in estimates with potential errors. A worrisome phenomenon is the alteration of V_d or metabolism with certain disease states. Examples are that the extrarenal clearance of cefotaxime, ciprofloxacin, piperacillin, phenobarbital, and theophylline decline with more severe illnesses and the variation in V_d widens. This is exacerbated by the duration of illness. Uremic substances or hepatically cleared substances may cause displacement from protein or tissue binding sites, altering PB and/or V_d. Edema increases the V_d

of aminoglycosides. These descriptions of altered pharmacokinetic parameters and the vagaries of drug–membrane interactions are reasons why predicting drug clearance/handling is fraught with uncertainty.

The third approach is described above and concluded with Equation 1. This approach utilizes the steady state plasma level, crudely determined by the plasma level obtained at the halfway point of the dosing interval.

The fourth approach ignores CRRT removal in that only total body clearance is addressed. This approach is the most precise in that drug levels will be determined and dosing adjustments made as clinical conditions alter total body clearance. CRRT is just one of the 'regional' clearances. Peak and trough plasma levels are needed and may be repeated until a pattern is established. The plasma level one desires must be known and will be termed the *desired level*. Generally the desired level is the targeted peak level. The *present level* is any level, but generally is the trough level. For a loading dose, the present level is zero. The *difference level* is the difference between the desired and the present levels. The **supplemental dose** is the dose needed to raise the present level to the desired level and is calculated by the following:

Equation 2   Supplemental dose = Difference level $\times$ V$_d$ $\times$ Body weight (kg)

This approach still suffers from errors between estimated V$_d$ and actual V$_d$, but with repeated sampling, this error is self-correcting. For drugs with the most concern for toxicity, levels are generally available.

Conclusions

Nothing is more descriptive of drug removal than actual data. Unfortunately, there are so many drugs and variations of CRRT operating conditions, that specific data do not always exist. The Bennett Tables recommendations are based on actual observations when such data exist, but the majority of dosing recommendations are based on theoretical extrapolation. This discussion should assist the clinician when data are lacking altogether.

In summary, dosing recommendations are based on actual clearance data, and when not available, on V$_d$ and PB. A V$_d$ of >0.6 is considered significant, decreasing CRRT removal. A PB of >80% suggests that much of the drug will not be removed. CRRTs are similar to high flux dialysis regarding the porosity of the extracorporeal membranes and similar in total solute clearance to a GFR about 15–20 ml/min. A day of CRRT is roughly equivalent to one hemodialysis treatment.

Index

Page numbers in *italic* indicate figures and tables.